THE OBESITY: Multiple Choice Questions

For

OBESITY BOARD EXAMINATION

REVIEW AND PREPARATION

FIFTH EDITION

VOLUME 1

Muhammad Asad MD

Author

Muhammad Asad MD, FACS, FASMBS

Bariatric and Minimally Invasive Surgeon

Diplomate American Board of Obesity Medicine

Contents

Table of Contents

Author	2
Contents	3
Preface	4
Contributors	5
Disclaimer	6
The Scope of The Problem	7
Etiology	23
Obesity – Relation with Other Diseases	71
Psychology and Counseling Aspects	108
Investigations for an Obese Patient	129
Principles of Dietary Management	177
Role of Physical Activity in Management of Obesity	223

Preface

The fifth edition of the Obesity Multiple Choice Questions book marks a milestone in the rapidly evolving field of obesity management. With increasing recognition among physicians and allied healthcare staff of the importance of addressing this critical health issue, the literature continues to expand, reflecting evolving recommendations and care standards. A regular update cycle ensures that the content remains relevant, serving as a problem-based learning tool for healthcare professionals.

In this iteration, the questions have been revamped, drawing inspiration from clinical cases to enrich the learning experience. A separate self-assessment exam opportunity is also available, providing an additional resource for thorough preparation.

This book isn't just another publication; it offers new perspectives and practical approaches that enhance the understanding of obesity management. It equips healthcare professionals with the essential tools and knowledge needed to effectively address this complex issue. The author's dedication and ongoing efforts are instrumental in advancing obesity management and improving healthcare education. Moreover, this book serves as an excellent tool for those preparing for the obesity board examination, offering comprehensive review materials and practical questions designed to help candidates succeed.

Muhammad Asad FACS, FASMBS
Diplomate American Board of Obesity Medicine

Contributors

Irtaza Asar
Attending Physician EM, Saint Vincent Hospital Erie, PA, USA
Hana Manzoor MD
Hospitalist, UPMC Hamot Erie, PA, USA

Disclaimer

© 2024 All rights reserved.

The book, in its entirety, may not be reproduced through any means, including written, electronic, recording, or photocopying, without obtaining written permission from the publisher or author. The only exceptions are brief quotations included in critical articles or reviews and specific pages where permissions have been granted.

While every effort has been taken to ensure the accuracy of the information within this book, the authors and publisher do not accept responsibility for any errors or omissions. The use of information from this publication is at the reader's discretion, and no liability is assumed for any resulting damages.

The Scope of The Problem

Question 1.1

Obesity has emerged as a significant health concern in recent times. Please choose the accurate statement.

a. The focus on reducing fat intake has resulted in a rise in carbohydrate consumption.
b. Food portions have increased significantly over the past few decades.
c. Lifestyle changes have led to a more sedentary way of living.
d. High-carbohydrate diets and the presence of insulin resistance are key factors contributing to substantial weight gain.
e. All of the above statements are correct.

The correct answer is "e."

In recent years, obesity has emerged as a significant health concern, affecting both developed and developing nations. Several key factors contribute to the development of obesity, including high carbohydrate diets, increased portion sizes, and sedentary lifestyles. Notably, individuals with insulin resistance are particularly susceptible to substantial weight gain when consuming high-carbohydrate foods.

Consuming just one regular soda daily can lead to a weight gain of approximately 10 to 15 pounds within a year. This highlights the significance of recognizing and addressing the dietary and lifestyle factors that contribute to obesity in our contemporary society. It emphasizes the need for making informed choices about beverage consumption and overall diet to maintain a healthy weight.

"Overweight & Obesity." Centers for Disease Control and Prevention, Centers for Disease Control and Prevention, 13 Aug. 2018, www.cdc.gov/obesity/data/adult.html.

Question 1.2

What is the prevalence of obesity in the US according to Statistics from the Center for Disease Control and Prevention (CDC))?

    a. 16.4%

    b. 19.4%

    c. 26.4%

    d. 31.4%

    e. 41.9%

The correct answer is "e."

The prevalence of obesity in the United States, according to statistics from the Center for Disease Control and Prevention (CDC), was approximately 41.9% of U.S. adults based on their Body Mass Index (BMI).

The prevalence of obesity among adults was 39.8% for those aged 20 to 39 years, 44.3% for those aged 40 to 59 years, and 41.5% for adults aged 60 and older.

https://www.cdc.gov/obesity/data/adult.html

Question 1.3

Which group of adults had the highest age-adjusted prevalence of obesity?
- a. Non-Hispanic White adults
- b. Non-Hispanic Asian adults
- c. Hispanic adults
- d. Non-Hispanic Black adults

The correct answer is "d."

The highest age-adjusted obesity prevalence was observed among Non-Hispanic Black adults (49.9%), followed by Hispanic adults (45.6%), Non-Hispanic White adults (41.4%), and Non-Hispanic Asian adults (16.1%).
https://www.cdc.gov/obesity/data/adult.html

5th Edition The Scope of The Problem

Question 1.4

A large study including analysis of data pooled from many prospective studies showed hazard ratio (HR) and BMI relationship among non-smokers with a simplified graph shown below.

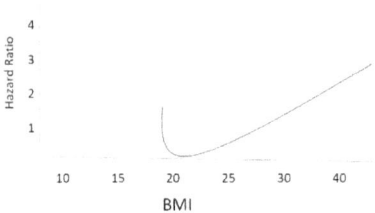

Figure (1)

Select the correct answer

    a. This graph shows an "S" shaped relationship

    b. The graph forms "J" shaped relationship

    c. The graph does not form "S" or "J" relationship

    d. The graph shows a symmetric "U" relationship

The correct answer is "b."

Question 1.5

Select the correct statement about additional information evident from this graph

　　a. Hazard ratio (HR) in BMI range of 25 to less than 30 is not increased

　　b. Hazard ratio (HR) in BMI range of 25 to less than 30 is decreased

　　c. There is a linear relationship between hazard ratio (HR) and BMI from BMI values 25 to 40

　　d. There is an inverse relationship between HR and BMI value up to around 40 BMI

The correct answer is "c."

The graph is a typical "J" shaped curve. There is a linear relationship between these two variables once BMI increases beyond 25 to 30.
Berrington de Gonzalez A. et al. N Engl J Med. 2010:363:2211-2219

Question 1.6

Recent prospective data from the United States has underscored a concerning rise in the relative risk of cancer-related mortality among individuals who are classified as obese. Among the list of cancers, which specific type demonstrates the most pronounced increase in mortality among those with a high BMI?

a. Cervical cancer
b. Uterine cancer
c. Pancreatic cancer
d. Renal cancer

The correct answer is "b."

It's crucial to highlight that the relative risk (RR) of cancer-related mortality is notably elevated in women when compared to men. Uterine cancer stands out with an exceptionally high RR of 6.25, followed by pancreatic cancer with an RR of 2.76, cervical cancer with an RR of 3.20, and renal carcinoma with an RR of 4.75. These statistics underscore the significance of comprehending the intricate connection between obesity and mortality from cancer.

Prospective Studies Collaboration, et al, Lancet. 2009: 373:1083-1096

Question 1.7

According to the American Medical Association Expert Committee recommendations, workup of obesity in children with comorbidities should include which of the following:

a. Lipid profile, liver profile, blood glucose, and kidney function tests for children above the 95th percentile

b. Only lipid profile and blood glucose tests for children above the 95th percentile

c. Lipid profile, liver profile, blood glucose, and kidney function tests for children between 80 to 85th percentile

d. Lipid profile, liver profile, blood glucose, and kidney function tests for children between 75th to 80th percentile

e. Lipid profile, liver profile, blood glucose, and kidney function tests are not recommended for children above the 85th percentile.

The correct answer is "a."

As per the guidelines from the American Medical Association Expert Committee on childhood obesity, the tests outlined in option "a" are essential components of the evaluation for obese children whose BMI exceeds the 95th percentile. It's worth emphasizing that kidney function assessments are included in the required profile for this specific percentile range. Notably, these tests yield valuable diagnostic information, particularly in patients falling within the 95th percentile and above.

Rao, G. Childhood obesity: highlights of AMA Expert Committee recommendations. Am Fam Physician. 2008;78:56-63.

Question 1.8
Which of the following statements about risk factors for development of Obstructive Sleep Apnea is incorrect?

    a. Neck circumference 17 inches and more for men

    b. Neck circumference 16 inches and more for women

    c. Younger obese people are more likely to have obstructive sleep apnea than older ones of similar weights.

    d. Upper body obesity

    e. An obese person with Mallampati's class 3

The correct answer is "c."

A neck circumference exceeding 40 cm (16 inches) for women and 43 cm (17 inches) for men with upper body obesity serves as a recognized risk factor for obstructive sleep apnea. Men face a greater risk compared to women, and advancing age also elevates the likelihood of developing obstructive sleep apnea.

The Mallampati score is a tool used in anesthesia to predict the ease of endotracheal intubation. This score assesses the visibility of specific oral cavity structures, such as the soft palate, uvula, and fauces, to gauge the potential difficulty of intubation. A high Mallampati score (class 3 or 4) indicates a more challenging intubation and is also associated with a higher risk of sleep apnea. The score is typically determined with the patient in a seated position, and it is a useful indirect indicator of intubation difficulty. However, for a more definitive assessment of intubation difficulty, the Cormack–Lehane classification system is used, which evaluates what is observed during direct laryngoscopy during the intubation process itself. There are variations in scoring based on the visibility of specific structures, and further research is needed to standardize Mallampati scoring effectively.

Flegal, K. M. (2002). Prevalence and Trends in Obesity Among US Adults, 1999-2000. Jama, 288(14), 1723-1727. doi:10.1001/jama.288.14.1723

Tucker, L. A., & Friedman, G. M. (1998). Obesity and Absenteeism: An Epidemiologic Study of 10,825 Employed Adults. American Journal of Health Promotion, 12(3), 202-207. doi:10.4278/0890-1171-12.3.202

May AL, Freedman D, Sherry B, Blanck H. Obesity - the United States, 1999-2010. MMWR Surveill Sum 2013;62(3): 120-128

https://en.wikipedia.org/wiki/Mallampati_scor

Question 1.9

Which of the following medical conditions is more common in the older age group of obese women compared to obese men?

    a. Diabetes Type 2

    b. Osteoarthrosis of the knees

    c. Obstructive Sleep Apnea

    d. Alzheimer's Disease

The correct answer is "d."

In the later stages of life, there is a notable association between obesity and an elevated risk of developing Alzheimer's dementia. This link is particularly pronounced among women, indicating that older women who are obese may be at a heightened risk of experiencing Alzheimer's disease. This underscores the significance of considering obesity as a potential risk factor for Alzheimer's, especially in the context of aging.

Gustafson, D., Rothenberg, E., Blennow, K., Steen, B., & Skoog, I. (2003). An 18-Year Follow-up of Overweight and Risk of Alzheimer Disease. Archives of Internal Medicine, 163(13), 1524-1528. doi:10.1001/archinte.163.13.1524

Question 1.10
Which class of obesity is assigned to a patient with BMI of 37?

   a. Overweight

   b. Class I obesity

   c. Class II obesity

   d. Class III obesity

The correct answer is "c."

BMI, or Body Mass Index, is a measure of weight relative to height, commonly used to assess weight categories. Here's a breakdown of BMI ranges and classifications:

Healthy BMI: 18.5 to 24.9

Overweight: 25 to 29.9

Class I Obesity: 30.0 to 34.9

Class II Obesity: 35 to 39.9

Class III Obesity: BMI value of 40 or higher

The World Health Organization (WHO) classifies weight categories into six groups, ranging from under-weight (BMI less than 18.5) to the categories mentioned above. Additionally, in some published surgical literature, a BMI of 50 or above is referred to as "super morbid obesity."The SuRF Report 2 (PDF). The Surveillance of Risk Factors Report Series (SuRF). World Health Organization. 2005. p. 22.

Question 1.11

In a family doctor's office, a husband and wife had their height and weight measured, and their body composition was assessed using a proprietary body fat analyzer. The reports revealed that the husband had a body fat percentage of 17%, while the wife had a body fat percentage of 33%. Please select the correct statement.

   a. The husband is likely to be an athlete.
   b. The husband is not obese.
   c. The wife has an acceptable body fat composition.
   d. The wife is identified as obese.

The correct answer is "d."

According to expert opinions, the following body fat percentage guidelines have been proposed.
Women with a body fat percentage of ≥ 32% and men with a body fat percentage of ≥ 25% are considered to be in the obesity range.
For women, body fat percentages between 25% and 31% and for men, between 18% and 24% are considered acceptable.
The fitness range is typically defined as 21% to 24% for women and 14% to 17% for men.
Athletes often have body fat percentages ranging from 14% to 20% for women and 6% to 13% for men.
It's worth noting that these figures have not been scientifically validated.
Author Natalie Digate Muth Health and Fitness Expert Natalie Digate Muth. "What Are the Guidelines for Percentage of Body Fat Loss?" ACE, www.acefitness.org/acefit/healthy-living-article/60/112/what-are-the-guidelines-for-percentage-of-body-fat.

Question 1.12

Which of the following statements is the most appropriate in advising the 25-year-old male who is undergoing a Bariatric program, engaging in heavy resistance exercises, and experiencing changes in his body composition without significant weight loss?

a. BMI remains as the best way to track his progress in future months.
b. BMI is more useful than % body fat (BF) to see his progress.
c. A more helpful tool may be % body fat.
d. % Body fat is not a very useful tool in this situation to monitor his progress.

The correct answer is "c."

% Body fat is considered a more suitable tool when there is an expected increase in muscle mass, as it provides a more accurate assessment of changes in body composition.

Question 1.13

Among the listed racial descents, which group has a higher risk for cardiovascular disease, type 2 diabetes, and the development of metabolic syndrome?

a. Japanese
b. Native Americans
c. South Asians
d. Scandinavians

The correct answer is "c."

Individuals of South Asian descent exhibit characteristics such as insulin resistance, elevated lipid levels, increased visceral fat, higher leptin levels, and elevated inflammatory cytokine levels compared to other populations. Due to these factors, their obesity criteria thresholds are set lower.

Holland, Ariel T., et al. "Spectrum of Cardiovascular Diseases in Asian-American Racial/Ethnic Subgroups." Annals of Epidemiology, vol. 21, no. 8, 2011, pp. 608–614., doi:10.1016/j.annepidem.2011.04.004.

Question 1.14

A 45-year-old male with a BMI of 32 kg/m² visits his primary care clinic for a routine check-up. During his visit, he expresses concerns about feeling judged due to his weight, which has deterred him from seeking medical care regularly. He is seeking advice on how to address weight stigma and improve his healthcare experience.

Which of the following strategies can healthcare providers implement to reduce weight stigma and improve the healthcare experience for patients with obesity?

a. Increase provider empathy through perspective-taking exercises and educate providers on the multifactorial causes of obesity.
b. Focus primarily on weight loss and frequent weigh-ins to emphasize the importance of reducing body weight.
c. Limit the use of specialized medical equipment to emphasize the need for patients to lose weight and fit standard equipment.
d. Encourage providers to avoid addressing obesity-related health risks to prevent patient discomfort.

The correct answer is "a."

Increasing provider empathy through perspective-taking exercises can help improve attitudes towards patients with obesity, making them feel more accepted and less judged. Educating providers on the genetic, environmental, biological, psychological, and social contributors to weight gain and loss fosters a more understanding and supportive approach. This strategy is aimed at creating a more welcoming and less threatening healthcare environment for patients with obesity, thereby improving their healthcare experience and adherence to medical advice. Other strategies include adopting patient-centered communication techniques and ensuring that the clinic environment accommodates patients of all sizes.

Phelan SM, Burgess DJ, Yeazel MW, Hellerstedt WL, Griffin JM, van Ryn M. Impact of weight bias and stigma on quality of care and outcomes for patients with obesity. Obes Rev. 2015 Apr;16(4):319-26. doi: 10.1111/obr.12266. Epub 2015 Mar 5. PMID: 25752756; PMCID: PMC4381543.

Etiology

Question 2.1

Which of the followings is the correct statement about etiology of obesity in the American population?

a. Substantial portion sizes

b. The increased popularity of Fast Food.

c. High energy but the lower nutrient density of food.

d. Low cost of processed food

e. All the above statements are correct.

The correct answer is "e."

The statements from "a." to "d." all appear to be accurate factors contributing to the development of obesity in the United States. Substantial portion sizes, coupled with the consumption of energy-rich diets, can indeed contribute to excessive calorie intake, which is a significant driver of obesity. Additionally, the affordability and widespread availability of processed foods that tend to be high in calories and low in nutritional value play a role in this complex issue. Addressing these factors is crucial in combating the obesity epidemic in the country.

Levian C, Ruiz E, Yang X. The pathogenesis of obesity from a genomic and systems biology perspective. Yale J Biol Med 2014; 87(2): 113–126

5th Edition Etiology

Question 2.2

Which of the following statements is true regarding the prevalence of obesity?

a. In the United States, the prevalence of obesity is more in higher socioeconomic segments of the population

b. In the United States, the prevalence of obesity is equal in both higher and lower socioeconomic segments of the population

c. In the United States, the prevalence of obesity is more in lower socioeconomic segments of the population

d. In developing countries, the prevalence of obesity is similar to the distribution of obesity seen in the United States

e. In developing countries, the prevalence of obesity is more in lower socioeconomic groups.

The correct answer is "c."

This fact reflects the specific challenges to lower socioeconomic groups where education, access to healthcare, and other resources are less as compared to more affluent segments of society.

Tillotson, J. E. (2004). AMERICAS OBESITY: Conflicting Public Policies, Industrial Economic Development, and Unintended Human Consequences. Annual Review of Nutrition, 24(1), 617-643. doi: 10.1146/annurev.nutr.24.012003.132434

Question 2.3

It is established that certain prenatal factors may increase the risk of developing obesity in later life. Which of the following statements is true?

a. Maternal malnutrition and diabetes can predispose an individual to develop diabetes and obesity in later life.

b. Low birth weight babies whose mothers have malnutrition in the first two trimesters are more prone to develop obesity in later life.

c. Smoking during pregnancy by mothers can increase the risk of obesity by several folds.

d. Breastfed babies are less prone to develop obesity as compared to bottle-fed infants.

e. All above statements are correct.

The correct answer is "e."

In recent years, several events related to the prenatal developmental phase and subsequent development of obesity have been recognized. Maternal malnutrition, diabetes, and smoking have been suggested as contributing factors for adult obesity. Historically, breastfeeding seemed to have a beneficial effect, but some studies appear to challenge this.

Lillycrop, K. A., & Burdge, G. C. (2010). Epigenetic changes in early life and future risk of obesity. International Journal of Obesity, 35(1), 72-83. doi:10.1038/ijo.2010.122

Question 2.4

Which of the following genotypes is related to the most common type of monogenic obesity?

a. Lipase hormone sensitive (LIPE) gene

b. Glucocorticoid receptor (NCR3C1) gene

c. G protein beta3 subunit (GNß3)

d. Melanocortin 4 receptor (MCR4) gene

e. Uncoupling protein 3 (UCP3)

The correct answer is "d."

Melanocortin 4 receptor deficiency runs in affected families. Salient features include early childhood obesity and hyperphagia. Metabolic workup shows insulin resistance, increased bone mineral density, and greater than expected linear growth. Gene polymorphism located at chromosome 18q22 is suggested.

Shriner D, et al. Genetic contributions to the development of obesity. In: Akabas S, Lederman S, Moore B, eds. Textbook of Obesity: Biological, Psychological, and Cultural Influences. West Sussex, UK: Wiley-Blackwell; 2012, pp. 79-86

Bays H, Scinta W: Adiposopathy and epigenetics: an introduction to obesity as a transgenerational disease. Curr Med Res Opin 2015 31:2059-2069.
10.1185/03007995.2015.1087983
https://www.ncbi.nlm.nih.gov/pubmed/26331354

Chung WK: An overview of monogenic and syndromic obesities in humans. Pediatr Blood Cancer 2012 58:122-128. 10.1002/pbc.23372
https://www.ncbi.nlm.nih.gov/pubmed/21994130

5th Edition Etiology

Question 2.5

Single gene mutations can lead to monogenic obesity. Select the correct answer regarding monogenic obesity.

    a. It is the most common form of obesity.

    b. It manifests in adult life.

    c. Affected genes belong primarily to the function of leptin-melanocortin pathways.

    d. Features of this kind of obesity include early onset, extreme obesity, increased food intake, and energy storage.

    e. "c." and "d." are correct.

The correct answer is "e."

Monogenic obesity is an uncommon form of obesity resulting from mutations in a single gene, which disrupts the regulation of appetite and metabolism. It typically emerges during childhood or adolescence and is frequently hereditary. Diagnosis entails genetic testing, and treatment approaches are tailored to the specific gene mutation, encompassing dietary adjustments, lifestyle modifications, or the potential use of pharmacological interventions.

Individuals affected by monogenic obesity experience extreme obesity. More than 1500 genes have been identified in relation to this condition. Examples include genes responsible for Leptin (LEP), Leptin receptor (LEPR), Proopiomelanocortin (POMC), and Melanocortin 4 receptor (MC4R).

Yale J, Levian C, Ruiz E, Yang X. The pathogenesis of obesity from a genomic and systems biology perspective. Biol Med 2014;87(2):113-26. eCollection 2014

5th Edition *Etiology*

Question 2.6

Which of the following is the most common human <u>obesity syndrome</u>?

    a. Bardet-Biedl syndrome

    b. Wilson-Turner syndrome

    c. Cohen syndrome

    d. Prader-Willi syndrome

    e. Börjeson-Forssman-Lehmann syndrome

The correct answer is "d."

Prader-Willi Syndrome stands as the most prevalent syndromic obesity disorder in humans. This syndrome encompasses a range of distinctive characteristics, including gradual weight accumulation, reduced fetal movement, muscle weakness (hypotonia), cognitive impairment, diminished stature, petite hands and feet, underdeveloped reproductive organs (hypogonadism), and an intense and insatiable appetite typically emerging between the first and second years of life.

Pérusse, L., Chagnon, Y. C., & Bouchard, C. (1998). Etiology of Massive Obesity: Role of Genetic Factors. World Journal of Surgery, 22(9), 907-912. doi:10.1007/s002689900493

Question 2.7
Regarding MC4R (Melanocortin 4 receptor) deficiency, which of the following statements is not correct?

 a. Heterozygous mutation is the most common monogenic form of obesity in childhood

 b. It is associated with early-onset obesity

 c. It is associated with shorter than average height

 d. Fasting insulin levels are high in patients with MC4R deficiency

The correct answer is "c."

Congenital deficiency of MC4R gene features obesity in both childhood and adult life. The onset of obesity is early and these patients are taller. High insulin levels may be contributory to the growth acceleration.

Savastano, D. M., Tanofsky-Kraff, M., Han, J. C., Ning, C., Sorg, R. A., Roza, C. A., . . . Yanovski, J. A. (2009). Energy intake and energy expenditure among children with polymorphisms of the melanocortin-3 receptor. American Journal of Clinical Nutrition, 90(4), 912-920. doi:10.3945/ajcn.2009.27537

Question 2.8

Which of the following syndromes is characterized by progressive obesity, diminished fetal activity, hypotonia after birth, mental retardation, short stature, behavioral abnormalities, hypogonadism, small hands, and feet, and hyperphagia?

    a. Bardet-Biedl syndrome

    b. Wilson-Turner syndrome

    c. Cohen syndrome

    d. Prader-Willi syndrome

    e. Börjeson-Forssman-Lehmann syndrome

The correct answer is "d."

Prader-Willi Syndrome is associated with hypotonia, stunted growth, mental retardation, short height, hypogonadism, hyperphagia, small hands and feet, and behavioral issues.

Question 2.9

Which of the following syndromes is characterized by polydactyly, developmental delay, impairment of vision, hypogonadism, central obesity, and renal abnormalities?

a. Bardet-Biedl syndrome

b. Wilson-Turner syndrome

c. Cohen syndrome

d. Prader-Willi syndrome

e. Börjeson-Forssman-Lehmann Syndrome

The correct answer is "a."

Bardet-Biedl syndrome results from an autosomal recessive gene mutation (BBS genes). Ciliary action of cells is affected. Defects in smell, vision, and hearing are seen in addition to abnormalities of chemical signals and cell movements.

Forsythe, Elizabeth, and Philip L Beales. "Bardet–Biedl Syndrome." European Journal of Human Genetics, vol. 21, no. 1, 2012, pp. 8–13., doi:10.1038/ejhg.2012.115.

5th Edition *Etiology*

Question 2.10

Select the correct statement regarding Gourmand syndrome.

a. Etiology is damage to the right frontal lobe.

b. The mechanism includes the loss of downstream satiety signaling from the hypothalamus.

c. These patients develop a new, post-injury passion for gourmet food.

d. All the above statements are correct.

The correct answer is "d."

This eating disorder is observed in individuals with impairment in the right anterior cerebral hemisphere. Moreover, alongside this condition, other impulse control disorders may coexist. It has been suggested that abnormalities in the serotonergic system may also play a role in the development of this disorder.

Regard, M., and Landis, T., "'Gourmand Syndrome': Eating Passion Associated with Right Anterior Lesions." Neurology, vol. 48, no. 5, Jan. 1997, pp. 1185–1190., doi:10.1212/wnl.48.5.1185.

Question 2.11
WAGR Obesity Syndrome is characterized by which of the following features?

    a. Wilms tumor

    b. Aniridia

    c. Genitourinary anomalies

    d. Mental retardation and obesity

    e. All the above

The correct answer is "e."

This syndrome involves a deletion mutation on chromosome 11 (11p13 region). Patients are predisposed to risk of developing Wilms tumor. Other features include abnormalities of the reproductive and urinary tracts. Intellectual disabilities are also seen.

Turleau, C., Grouchy, J. D., Nihoul-Fékété, C., Dufier, J. L., Chavin-Colin, F., & Junien, C. (1984). Del11p13/nephroblastoma without aniridia. Human Genetics, 67(4), 455-456. doi:10.1007/bf00291410

Question 2.12

In the context of craniopharyngiomas, all the statements below are true with one exception.

    a. It is a rare hypothalamic tumor that leads to obesity.

    b. It is characterized by peak incidence rates at ages 5-15 and 50-60 years.

    c. Hyperinsulinemia and leptin resistance is seen in these patients.

    d. Reduced sympathetic tone leads to low physical activity and low metabolic rate.

    e. Surgical resection of the hypothalamus is mostly curative.

The correct answer is "e."

Statements "a.," "b., "c.," and "d." are correct. Surgery is not always curative. Tumor recurrence is high in the initial years. In instances of subtotal removal, the 5-year disease free rate is 48.3%.

"Craniopharyngioma." Wikipedia, Wikimedia Foundation, 11 Aug. 2018, en.wikipedia.org/wiki/Craniopharyngioma.

5th Edition Etiology

Question 2.13

A hormone has the following characteristics.

1. Its level increases during diet induced weight loss
2. Its level increases with sleep deprivation
3. It mediates the sense of hunger.
4. IV administration decreases fat oxidation and increases food intake with adiposity.

Which of the following hormones has the features stated above?

- a. Ghrelin
- b. Leptin
- c. Testosterone
- d. Thyroid hormone
- e. Growth hormone

The correct answer is "a."

Ghrelin is a hormone produced by the gastrointestinal (GI) tract, specifically in the stomach lining. It functions as one of the neuropeptides involved in regulating appetite and energy balance within the body. Ghrelin is often referred to as the "hunger hormone" because it stimulates appetite and plays a role in maintaining energy homeostasis by influencing metabolism and energy storage.

Kojima, M., Hosoda, H., Date, Y., Nakazato, M., Matsuo, H., & Kangawa, K. (1999). Ghrelin is a growth-hormone-releasing acylated peptide from stomach. Nature, 402(6762), 656-660. doi:10.1038/45230

5th Edition Etiology

Question 2.14

In the context of the central nervous system's regulation of hunger, which of the following is not an anorexigen (a substance that suppresses appetite)?

a. POMC (proopiomelanocortin)

b. α-MSH (α-Melanocyte-stimulating hormone)

c. CART (cocaine-and amphetamine-regulated transcript)

d. NPY (neuropeptide Y)

The correct answer is "d."

Neuropeptide Y is a neuropeptide found in the mammalian nervous system. It has a dual role in promoting food intake and facilitating fat storage. Moreover, it plays a significant role in managing anxiety, stress, and pain. In contrast, all the other options mentioned earlier have anorexigenic effects, meaning they suppress appetite.

Decressac, M., & Barker, R. (2012). Neuropeptide Y and its role in CNS disease and repair. Experimental Neurology, 238(2), 265-272. doi: 10.1016/j.expneurol.2012.09.004

Question 2.15
Which of the following neurohormones is not an orexigen (stimulators of hunger)?

    a. NPY (Neuropeptide Y)

    b. Agouti Related Peptide (AgRP)

    c. Serotonin

    d. MCH (Melanin-concentrating hormone)

The correct answer is "c."

Serotonin is an appetite suppressant. More than 80 percent of the body's serotonin is produced in GI tract. Serotonin is also produced in the brain. It does affect mood and emotional energy. Carbohydrate consumption can influence serotonin levels in the brain, potentially leading to temporary mood improvement and appetite control. However, the relationship is complex and can vary among individuals, and long-term dietary choices should be made with consideration of overall health.

Question 2.16

Neuropeptide Y (NPY) plays a significant role in hunger and weight maintenance. Select the correct statement regarding this hormone.

a. It increases food intake (orexigenic)
b. It promotes storage of fat.
c. Stimulated by Ghrelin
d. In obese patients elevated levels of NPY are seen
e. All the above statements are correct.

The correct answer is "e."

Overall, NPY is a multifaceted neuropeptide that contributes to various physiological processes in the body, including the regulation of appetite, energy balance, fat storage, and cell growth. Its presence in specific brain regions underscores its significance in coordinating these functions. However, dysregulation of NPY levels can also be associated with certain health conditions, such as obesity and stress-related disorders.

Schwartz, M. W. (1992). Inhibition of hypothalamic neuropeptide Y gene expression by insulin. Endocrinology, 130(6), 3608-3616. doi:10.1210/en.130.6.3608

Question 2.17

Regarding AgRP (Agouti Related Peptide), which of the following statements is not correct?

a. It is an orexigenic chemical.
b. Found in first-order neurons in arcuate nucleus.
c. Keeps hunger from turning down.
d. Acts on MC3R and MC4R receptors on second-order neurons to block effects of ROMC/CART (α-MSH)
e. It is primarily an anorexigenic hormone.

The correct answer is "e."

Agouti-related protein (AgRP) is a neuropeptide produced in the brain, specifically in the arcuate nucleus of the hypothalamus. It plays a crucial role in the regulation of appetite, energy balance, and body weight.
Here are key points about Agouti-related protein (AgRP):
Appetite Regulation
AgRP is often referred to as an "orexigenic" peptide, meaning it stimulates appetite. When AgRP is released in the brain, it promotes feelings of hunger and the desire to eat. This effect is part of a complex neural network that controls when and how much we eat.
Counterpart to Melanocortins
AgRP works in opposition to another group of neuropeptides called melanocortins. Melanocortins, including alpha-melanocyte-stimulating hormone (α-MSH), reduce appetite and increase energy expenditure. AgRP, on the other hand,

inhibits the activity of melanocortin receptors, leading to an increase in appetite and a decrease in energy expenditure.

Role in Energy Balance

AgRP is part of the body's regulatory system for maintaining energy balance. When energy stores in the body are low (e.g., during fasting or calorie restriction), AgRP levels may increase to stimulate food intake and conserve energy. Conversely, when energy stores are sufficient, melanocortins predominate to suppress appetite and promote energy expenditure.

Complex Neural Circuitry

The regulation of appetite and energy balance is a complex process involving multiple neuropeptides and neural pathways. AgRP is just one component of this intricate system, working in concert with other factors like leptin (a hormone produced by fat cells) and the melanocortin system.

Relevance to Obesity Research

Research on AgRP has provided valuable insights into the molecular and neural mechanisms underlying obesity and appetite control. Dysregulation of AgRP and its interactions with other appetite-regulating peptides can contribute to obesity and related metabolic disorders.

Jackson, P.J. et al. (2006) Structural and molecular evolutionary analysis of Agouti and Agouti-related proteins. Chem. Biol. 13, 1297–1305

Question 2.18

Orexin and MCH (melanocyte-concentrating hormone) are neurohormones. Which of the following statements is not correct?

a. These are orexigenic chemicals.

b. Found in second-order neurons in the lateral hypothalamus.

c. These hormones are anorexigenic.

d. They act on higher order neurons to stimulate arousal, anxiety, aggression, feeding, pleasure, reward, and learning.

The correct answer is "c."

Orexin and MCH both have a role in sleep regulation and are considered to be orexigenic.

Delgado, J.M. and Anand, B.K. (1953) "Increase of food intake induced by electrical stimulation of the lateral hypothalamus," The American Journal of Physiology. 172 (1): 162–168.

Question 2.19

Which of the following statements is not correct regarding proopiomelanocortin (POMC)?

a. It is an anorexigenic hormone.
b. It is found in first-order neurons in arcuate nucleus.
c. It releases α- MSH which acts on second-order neuron MC3R and MC4R receptors.
d. It is orexigenic in nature.

The correct answer is "d."

Proopiomelanocortin (POMC) is a precursor protein found in various body tissues, producing vital peptides like α-MSH and ACTH. These peptides influence functions such as pigmentation, cortisol production, and appetite regulation. POMC-derived α-MSH acts as an appetite suppressant by stimulating the hypothalamus, responding to nutrient and leptin levels. Dysregulation in the POMC system can contribute to obesity.

Question 2.20

Which of the following statements is not correct regarding cocaine-and amphetamine-regulated transcript (CART)?

a. It is anorexigenic in nature.

b. It is found with NPY in arcuate nucleus or alone in lateral hypothalamus.

c. Its mechanism of action may involve the central release of GLP-1

d. It is orexigenic in nature.

The correct answer is "d."

CART hypoactivity in the hypothalamus causes hyperphagia and weight gain in experimental animals.

Nakhate, K. T., Kokare, D. M., Singru, P. S., & Subhedar, N. K. (2010). Central regulation of feeding behavior during social isolation of rat: evidence for the role of endogenous CART system. International Journal of Obesity, 35(6), 773-784. doi:10.1038/ijo.2010.231

5th Edition Etiology

Question 2.21

Select the correct statement regarding leptin.

a. It is an anorexigenic in nature.

b. It is primarily produced by white adipose tissue.

c. Its mechanism of action involves direct stimulation of POMC/CART, turns off GABA inhibition of POMC and inhibits orexin.

d. Its mechanism of action involves inhibition of NPY/AgRP

e. All above statements are correct.

The correct answer is "e."

Leptin is a hormone produced by fat cells that plays a crucial role in regulating appetite, metabolism, and body weight. Leptin serves as a key player in regulating food intake through a multifaceted communication system involving the gut, adipose tissue, and the brain. It is secreted by adipose tissue following meals, signaling fullness by binding to hypothalamic receptors. This mechanism controls short-term food intake, with breakfast triggering a satiety response.

Additionally, leptin influences long-term food intake and fat storage. The magnitude and duration of post-meal satiety are determined by the amount of adipose tissue available to produce leptin. Dieting reduces both adipose tissue mass and post-meal leptin levels, leading to a gradual decline in the satiety response and increased food intake until baseline levels are restored. This phenomenon explains the common occurrence of weight regain after dieting.

Question 2.22

Select the incorrect statement regarding leptin deficiency.

a. It is the most common form of obesity in humans.

b. Affected individuals are affected in early childhood.

c. Leptin levels are high in patients with leptin receptor defects.

d. Puberty is delayed and hypogonadism is seen in affected individuals.

The correct answer is "a."

Leptin deficiency is an exceedingly rare genetic condition characterized by the absence or severe reduction of the hormone leptin, which is typically produced by fat tissue. This condition leads to early-onset and extreme obesity due to uncontrolled appetite and disrupted appetite regulation. In addition to obesity, individuals with leptin deficiency may experience metabolic abnormalities. The primary treatment involves leptin replacement therapy, aiming to restore normal appetite control and metabolic function. Leptin deficiency is exceptionally rare, and most cases of obesity result from a complex interplay of genetic, environmental, and lifestyle factors.

Kelesidis, T. (2010). Narrative Review: The Role of Leptin in Human Physiology: Emerging Clinical Applications. Annals of Internal Medicine, 152(2), 93-100. doi:10.7326/0003-4819-152-2-201001190-00008

5th Edition Etiology

Question 2.23
Which of the following statements is true?

a. Testosterone levels and insulin resistance have an inverse relationship.

b. PPAR-α (peroxisome proliferator-activated receptor alpha) is active under conditions of excess energy.

c. Growth hormone deficiency increases lean body mass.

d. Hyperthyroidism may cause fluid retention, decreased metabolism, and weight gain.

e. Growth hormone excess increases visceral fat mass

The correct answer is "a."

Testosterone levels and insulin resistance share an inverse relationship with each other. Growth hormones lead to increased lean body mass. Hypothyroidism can cause fluid retention and weight gain. Growth hormones cause a decrease in visceral fat mass. PPAR-α is active in situations of energy deprivation.

Question 2.24

A young female presents with central obesity, insulin resistance, hyperinsulinemia, diabetes, and excessive hair growth on the face. Select the correct statement.

a. This patient is unlikely to have infertility.

b. Insulin level is likely to be low.

c. Lipoprotein lipase is expected to be more active.

d. Menstrual periods are expected to be unaffected.

e. Metformin is contraindicated in these cases.

The correct answer is "c."

The characteristics described above are indicative of a typical presentation of polycystic ovarian syndrome (PCOS). Commonly observed symptoms include infertility, elevated insulin levels, and irregular menstrual cycles. Metformin is a frequently prescribed medication for managing this condition. Lipoprotein lipase is an enzyme responsible for storing fat and can contribute to increased visceral fat accumulation. In younger girls who have recently started menstruating, cyclic menstrual irregularities may be observed. In some cases, a period of initial observation without specific treatment may be considered appropriate.

Jensen MD. Obesity. In: Goldman L, Schafer A, eds. Cecil Textbook of Medicine, 24th ed. Philadelphia, PA: Saunders Elsevier; 2012, pp. 1409-17.

Question 2.25

A hormone has the following features.

1. It is derived from fat

2. It is anorexigenic

3. It reduces food intake

4. Its levels are increased in obesity

Which of the following hormones is discussed above?

    a. Ghrelin

    b. Testosterone

    c. Growth hormone

    d. Leptin

    e. Insulin

The correct answer is "d."

Leptin is the hormone with features stated above.

O'rourke, R. W. (2014). Metabolic Thrift and the Genetic Basis of Human Obesity. Annals of Surgery, 259(4), 642-648. doi:10.1097/sla.0000000000000361

5th Edition Etiology

Question 2.26

Which of the following statements is correct regarding adipocytes?

a. Lipoprotein lipase is involved in fat elaboration and released from adipocytes.

b. Hormone-sensitive lipase is involved in storing fat.

c. Adiponectin is the most abundant adipokine in fat.

d. Adiponectin levels are increased during obesity.

e. Adipocytes do not play a significant role in the outcomes of obesity.

The correct answer is "c."

Adiponectin stands as the predominant adipokine within fat cells, contributing to heightened insulin sensitivity and mitigating the effects triggered by tumor necrosis factor-alpha (TNF-α). In contrast, lipoprotein lipase plays a role in fat storage, while hormone-sensitive lipase is responsible for the breakdown and release of fat from adipocytes.

Racette SB, Deusinger SS, Deusinger RH. Obesity: Overview of prevalence, etiology, and treatment. Phys Ther. 2003;83(3): 276-88

5th Edition Etiology

Question 2.27
Which of the following statements is correct regarding the influence of psychological factors in the development of obesity?

a. Restraint disinhibition may be a critical factor in the etiology of obesity.

b. History of sexual abuse during childhood can lead to the development of obesity in later life.

c. Binge eating disorder involves the consumption of a significant amount of food in 2 hours period characterized by a feeling of loss of control. It is estimated in up to 50% of cases who seek bariatric surgery.

d. Night eating disorder involves the consumption of up to 25% of one's daily caloric intake during the evening and night. It happens at least two times per week for at least three months.

e. All above are correct.

The correct answer is "e."

Here choices "a," to "d." are all correct. It is recognized that restraint disinhibition, history of sexual abuse in childhood, binge eating, and night eating disorders contribute to the development of obesity.

In binge eating disorder patients consume a large quantity of food more than once every week for the last three months. It is identified in 2-3 percent of the adult population in the United States. More than half of patients with severe obesity are thought to have this eating disorder. Patients do not show behaviors like purging or excessive exercise. Lisdexamfetamine has been found to be useful in the treatment of this disorder. This medicine is a Schedule II drug. This drug has the potential for abuse and dependence.

Redinger, R. N. (2008). The Prevalence and Etiology of Nongenetic Obesity and Associated Disorders. Southern Medical Journal, 101(4), 395-399. doi: 10.1097/01.smj.0000308879.67271.09nia

Etiology

Question 2.28

Which of the following statements is true for the etiology of development of obesity?

a. Overweight individuals have low levels of C-reactive proteins.

b. Different microorganisms have been studied as possible etiologies of obesity. Avian adenovirus SMAM-1 and human adenovirus Ad-36 have been suspected to have a link to develop obesity.

c. The gut microbiome is not linked to the development of obesity.

d. Most children who tested positive for Ad-36 are not likely to be obese.

e. All above are correct.

The correct answer is "b."

C-reactive protein levels are elevated in individuals with obesity, and there is substantial evidence supporting the connection between the gut microbiome and the development of obesity. Additionally, various viruses are under investigation for their potential involvement in the development of obesity.

Atkinson, R. L. (2007). Viruses as an Etiology of Obesity. Mayo Clinic Proceedings, 82(10), 1192-1198. doi:10.4065/82.10.1192

Question 2.29

Which of the following statements is true regarding eating behaviors?

　　a. Having a regular breakfast routine may help prevent obesity.

　　b. People consuming more than 33% of the daily intake of energy in the evening are twice as likely to have obesity.

　　c. Fat storage tendency of the body is increased during late evening hours.

　　d. Caffeine, ethanol, and sodium may alter circadian rhythms and can have a possible role in the development of obesity.

　　e. All the above statements are correct.

The correct answer is "e."

Consistently having breakfast appears to be beneficial in preventing weight gain. Conversely, late-night eating poses a risk factor for obesity due to the altered hormonal dynamics during nighttime. Similarly, excessive consumption of caffeine and alcohol may also play a role in contributing to weight gain.

5th Edition *Etiology*

Question 2.30

Which of the following statements is true regarding eating behaviors?

a. High calcium in the diet increases the risk of gaining weight by inhibiting metabolic pathways.

b. Fast eaters are less likely to be obese.

c. Consumption of some vitamins like niacin and vitamin C can promote obesity.

d. Regularly consuming high-protein and high-fat foods, such as cheese, may not be a substantial contributing factor to the development of obesity

e. None of the above statements is true

The correct answer is "c."

Niacin (B3) has been reported to have a stimulating effect. Additionally, high doses of B1 and B2 have been associated with the development of obesity. Vitamin C, in excessive amounts, can adversely affect reactive oxygen element levels and potentially lead to weight gain. Furthermore, the consumption of substantial quantities of full-fat cheese can also contribute to weight gain.

Zhou, S. (2014). Excess vitamin intake: An unrecognized risk factor for obesity. World J Diabetes, 5(1), 1. doi:10.4239/wjd.V5.i1.1

Question 2.31

Which of the following statements concerning the consumption of sugar in liquid form as opposed to solid form is accurate?

    a. Gastric emptying and transit time increases

    b. Reduced postprandial ghrelin suppression

    c. Increased postprandial hunger

    d. Larger calorie intake in subsequent meals

    e. All above statements are correct

The correct answer is "e."

Liquid sugars have several effects, including accelerated stomach emptying, reduced suppression of post-meal ghrelin, and heightened post-meal hunger, potentially leading to increased consumption in subsequent meals.

Dimeglio, D., & Mattes, R. (2000). Liquid versus solid carbohydrate: effects on food intake and body weight. International Journal of Obesity, 24(6), 794-800. doi: 10.1038/sj.ijo.0801229

Question 2.32

Resting energy expenditure and non-exercise activity thermogenesis play a crucial role in both the health and the development of obesity. Which of the following statements is accurate?

a. Resting energy expenditure accounts for 15 to 20% of daily energy expenditure.

b. Individuals residing in Arctic regions are more prone to having a lower BMR (basal metabolic rate).

c. BMR exhibits an inverse relationship with lean body mass.

d. Adding an additional hour of sitting per day, compared to standing, could result in approximately 6 pounds of weight gain annually.

e. Energy-restricted diets are unlikely to significantly alter BMI (Body Mass Index.

The correct answer is "d."

There is substantial evidence supporting the negative consequences of sedentary lifestyles. Resting energy expenditure typically constitutes 60 to 70% of total energy expenditure. Individuals with greater lean body mass are anticipated to exhibit higher BMR. Colder weather conditions can result in increased calorie expenditure.

Weinsier, RL, Hunter, GR, Heini, AF, Goran, MI, Sell, SM. (1998) The etiology of obesity relative contribution of metabolic factors, diet, and physical activity. Am J Med. 105(2),145-50.

Question 2.33

Which of the following statements is true regarding Thermic Effect of Food (TEF), Non-Exercise Activity Thermogenesis (NEAT) and Physical Activity (PA)?

a. Approximately 20% of TEF is obligatory (digestion, absorption, and storage of nutrients) and 80 % is facultative thermogenesis.

b. TEF is higher in insulin-resistant obese individuals.

c. Lower levels of NEAT may predict future weight gain.

d. Epidemiologically, the role of PA in obesity and weight gain is less consistent than the role of energy intake to the development of obesity.

e. None of the above statements is true.

The correct answer is "c."

60 to 70 % of the thermic effect of meals is obligatory, and the remaining 30 to 40 % is facultative thermogenesis. Lower levels of NEAT can contribute to weight gain.

Tappy, L. (1996). Thermic effect of food and sympathetic nervous system activity in humans. Reproduction Nutrition Development, 36(4), 391-397. doi:10.1051/rnd:19960405

Weinsier, RL, Hunter, GR, Heini, AF, Goran, MI, Sell, SM. (1998) The etiology of obesity relative contribution of metabolic factors, diet, and physical activity. Am J Med. 105(2),145-50.

Question 2.34

Energy homeostasis plays a vital role in weight maintenance and comprises several components. Among them, "Basal Metabolic Rate" (BMR) and "Physical Activity" (PA) are particularly significant. Which of the following statements is accurate?

a. Basal metabolic rate constitutes approximately 20 to 30% of total body expenditure of energy.
b. Basal metabolic rate constitutes approximately 60 to 70 % of total body expenditure of energy.
c. Physical activity accounts for 60 to 70% of total body expenditure of energy.
d. Physical activity accounts for 40 to 50% of total body expenditure of energy.

The correct answer is "b."

60 to 70 percent of body energy is spent by BMR. Physical activity is one of the most modifiable factors.

Question 2.35

A 22-year-old female presents with obesity, having a BMI of 38. Her height is approximately 55 inches (140 cm), and she exhibits a rounded face. An oral examination reveals poorly developed teeth. Additionally, deformities are observed in her hands and feet. X-rays of her hands indicate short fourth metacarpals, along with deformities in other short bones. Her calcium level is 6.6 mg/dl, and phosphate is low. A genetic cause is suspected. Please choose the correct diagnosis.

a. Prader-Willi syndrome
b. Albright's hereditary osteodystrophy
c. Cohen syndrome
d. Down's syndrome

The correct answer is "b."

The presented features in this case point towards Albright's hereditary osteodystrophy, which is associated with a G protein abnormality caused by a defective GNAS1 gene. In contrast, Cohen syndrome is attributed to an autosomal recessive gene mutation in VPS13B (COH1 gene). Cohen syndrome is characterized by developmental delay, retinal abnormalities, thick eyebrows and eyelashes, hypotonia, ligament laxity, lower IQ, and a smaller head size.

Bays H, Scinta W: Adiposopathy and epigenetics: an introduction to obesity as a transgenerational disease. Curr Med Res Opin 2015 31:2059-2069.
10.1185/03007995.2015.1087983
https://www.ncbi.nlm.nih.gov/pubmed/26331354

5th Edition Etiology

Question 2.36

Which of the following statements best describes the role of peripheral serotonin in energy balance and lipid metabolism?

a. Peripheral serotonin increases lipid absorption and storage by promoting fat deposition and lipogenesis in the liver, insulin release in the pancreas, and inhibiting thermogenesis in brown adipose tissue (BAT).
b. Peripheral serotonin decreases lipid absorption and storage by inhibiting fat deposition and lipogenesis in the liver, reducing insulin release in the pancreas, and promoting thermogenesis in brown adipose tissue (BAT).
c. Peripheral serotonin has no significant effect on lipid absorption and storage, and its primary role is limited to modulating gut motility and vasodilation.
d. Peripheral serotonin exclusively increases thermogenesis in brown adipose tissue (BAT) and browning of white adipose tissue (WAT), leading to reduced lipid storage.

The correct answer is "a."

Peripheral serotonin synthesized by enterochromaffin (EC) cells in response to luminal nutrients plays a significant role in promoting lipid absorption and storage. It facilitates fat deposition and lipogenesis in the liver, enhances insulin release in the pancreas which further increases adipogenesis and lipogenesis, and inhibits BAT thermogenesis and browning of WAT. These actions collectively contribute to efficient lipid storage, highlighting serotonin's role as a key modulator of energy balance.

Understanding peripheral serotonin's impact on nutrient absorption, storage, and utilization in specific tissues is crucial. The development of tissue-selective Tph1 and HTR knockout mice will help clarify serotonin's complex signaling network. This research could lead to new treatments for metabolic diseases like obesity, type 2 diabetes, and NAFLD by targeting these pathways.

Yabut JM, Crane JD, Green AE, Keating DJ, Khan WI, Steinberg GR. Emerging Roles for Serotonin in Regulating Metabolism: New Implications for an Ancient Molecule. Endocr Rev. 2019 Aug 1;40(4):1092-1107. doi: 10.1210/er.2018-00283. PMID: 30901029; PMCID: PMC6624793.

5th Edition Etiology

Question 2.37

Which of the following statements about the role of various chemicals in obesity is correct?

   a. Dibutyltin (DBT) is a breakdown product of tributyltin (TBT) and has been shown to induce adipogenesis and insulin resistance in animal studies.
   b. Bisphenol A analogues, such as BPS and BPF, are completely safe alternatives to BPA and do not contribute to obesity in any age group.
   c. Acrylamide exposure has been found to consistently reduce the risk of obesity in both animal and human studies.
   d. Dioctyl sodium sulfosuccinate (DOSS) has no impact on adipogenesis or the development of obesity in animal models.

The correct answer is "a."

Dibutyltin (DBT) has been demonstrated to promote adipogenesis and cause insulin resistance in animal models, indicating its role as an obesogen. Bisphenol A (BPA) analogues, such as BPS and BPF, have been linked to obesity in children and may still pose risks, making them not completely safe alternatives. Acrylamide's association with obesity is inconsistent, with some studies showing positive associations with biomarkers of obesity and others showing no or negative associations. Dioctyl sodium sulfosuccinate (DOSS) has been shown to induce adipogenesis and promote obesity in animal models, particularly when exposure occurs during the perinatal period.

Egusquiza RJ, Blumberg B. Environmental Obesogens and Their Impact on Susceptibility to Obesity: New Mechanisms and Chemicals. Endocrinology. 2020 Mar 1;161(3):bqaa024. doi: 10.1210/endocr/bqaa024. PMID: 32067051; PMCID: PMC7060764.

5th Edition Etiology

Question 2.38

Growth differentiation factor 15 (GDF-15), part of the transforming growth factor beta superfamily, has been recognized as a crucial mediator of the weight loss effects induced by metformin. Which of the following statements best describes the mechanism of GDF-15 in reducing food intake and body weight?

   a. GDF-15 binds to the GFRAL receptor, which is widely expressed in various tissues, leading to a decrease in food intake and body weight.
   b. GDF-15 binds exclusively to the GFRAL receptor in the brainstem, forming a complex with the coreceptor RET, which activates a neuronal network to reduce food intake and body weight.
   c. GDF-15 binds to multiple receptors in the brain, reducing food intake and body weight through various signaling pathways.
   d. GDF-15 acts directly on adipose tissue to reduce fat accumulation and body weight.

The correct answer is "b."

The weight-related effect of GDF-15 relies on its interaction with the GFRAL receptor and the coreceptor RET. GFRAL, primarily expressed in the brainstem, was validated as the sole high-affinity ligand for GDF-15. Activation of GFRAL by GDF-15 stimulates a neuronal network that reduces food intake and appetite. GFRAL knockout mice do not experience the weight loss and reduced food intake effects of GDF-15, demonstrating GFRAL's essential role. Additionally, the signaling cascade triggered by GDF-15 involves GFRAL and RET interaction, with the ERK pathway playing a significant role. Blocking RET can prevent GDF-15-mediated signaling.

Ouyang J, Isnard S, Lin J, Fombuena B, Peng X, Chen Y, Routy JP. GDF-15 as a Weight Watcher for Diabetic and Non-Diabetic People Treated With Metformin. Front Endocrinol (Lausanne). 2020 Nov 18;11:581839. doi: 10.3389/fendo.2020.581839. PMID: 33312159; PMCID: PMC7708317.

5th Edition *Etiology*

Question 2.39
Which of the following mechanisms best explains how obesity-associated inflammation in skeletal muscle contributes to insulin resistance?

a. Enhanced fatty acid oxidation in myocytes
b. Increased polarization of immune cells into proinflammatory phenotypes in intermuscular adipose tissue (IMAT) and perimuscular adipose tissue (PMAT)
c. Decreased secretion of proinflammatory molecules from adipose tissue
d. Increased synthesis of anti-inflammatory cytokines in skeletal muscle

The correct answer is "b."

Accumulating evidence indicates that obesity is associated with increased inflammation in skeletal muscle (SM), primarily due to enhanced immune cell infiltration in intermuscular adipose tissue (IMAT) and perimuscular adipose tissue (PMAT). This inflammatory infiltration includes an increased presence of immune cells that tend to polarize into proinflammatory phenotypes. These cells express elevated levels of proinflammatory molecules, which, along with inflammatory molecules from other tissues, especially adipose tissue (AT), negatively regulate myocyte metabolic functions. This regulation contributes to local insulin resistance in skeletal muscle and systemic insulin resistance throughout the body.

Options a., c., and d. are incorrect because they do not accurately describe the mechanisms by which obesity-related inflammation contributes to insulin resistance. Enhanced fatty acid oxidation (option a.) is not typically associated with increased inflammation. Decreased secretion of proinflammatory molecules from adipose tissue (option c.) would likely reduce, rather than contribute to, insulin resistance. Increased synthesis of anti-inflammatory cytokines in skeletal muscle (option d.) would also reduce inflammation and is not a characteristic of obesity-related inflammation. Wu H, Ballantyne CM. Skeletal muscle inflammation and insulin resistance in obesity. J Clin Invest. 2017 Jan 3;127(1):43-54. doi: 10.1172/JCI88880. Epub 2017 Jan 3. PMID: 28045398; PMCID: PMC5199705.

Question 2.40

A patient presents with a history of chronic overeating and difficulty in weight management. Investigations reveal altered activity in hypothalamic neurons associated with feeding behavior. Specifically, AgRP neurons demonstrate reduced suppression of activity despite calorie intake, suggesting a lack of appropriate signaling in response to caloric consumption. This patient is likely experiencing dysregulation in which of the following pathways or systems?

   a. Dysfunction in AgRP neuron plasticity
   b. Reduced synaptic plasticity in proopiomelanocortin (POMC) neurons
   c. Increased activation of the caudal nucleus of the solitary tract (NTS)
   d. Enhanced feedback from orbitofrontal cortex (OFC) affecting motivational state

The correct answer is "a." The patient exhibits signs of improper suppression of AgRP neuron activity following caloric intake, a key characteristic in the regulation of feeding behavior and energy homeostasis. Dysfunction in AgRP neuron plasticity could lead to impaired feedback mechanisms, resulting in the described symptoms. Other options, such as reduced POMC neuron plasticity, activation of the NTS, or influence from the OFC, do not directly explain the specific lack of suppression in AgRP neuron activity despite caloric intake.

Su Z, Alhadeff AL, Betley JN. Nutritive, post-ingestive signals are the primary regulators of AgRP neuron activity. *Cell Rep*. 2017; **21**(10): 2724-2736.

Obesity – Relation with Other Diseases

Question 3.1

Which of the following statements regarding the relation of obesity to other diseases is correct?

a. Higher prevalence of cancer-related fatalities is observed among obese individuals with malignancies affecting the colon, rectum, gallbladder, liver, pancreas, kidney, esophagus, myelomas, and certain lymphomas.

b. Osteoarthrosis risk increases by three folds in people with BMI more than 27.

c. Non-alcoholic fatty liver disease (NAFLD) may affect up to 70 percent of patients with type 2 diabetes mellitus.

d. Prevalence of major depression increases to almost four times once BMI exceeds from 25 to 35.

e. All the above statements are correct.

The correct answer is "e."

The incidence of various cancers and related mortality is higher in the obese population. Other disorders like osteoarthrosis, fatty liver disease, and depression also occur at an increased frequency.

Wright, M. E., Chang, S., Schatzkin, A., Albanes, D., Kipnis, V., Mouw, T., . . . Leitzmann, M. F. (2007). Prospective study of adiposity and weight change in relation to prostate cancer incidence and mortality. Cancer, 109(4), 675-684. doi:10.1002/cncr.22443

Reijman, M., Pols, H. A., Bergink, A. P., Hazes, J. M., Belo, J. N., Lievense, A. M., & Bierma-Zeinstra, S. M. (2006). Body mass index associated with onset and progression of osteoarthritis of the knee but not of the hip: The Rotterdam Study. Annals of the Rheumatic Diseases, 66(2), 158-162. doi:10.1136/ard.2006.053538

Adams, L. A. (2006). Treatment of non-alcoholic fatty liver disease. Postgraduate Medical Journal, 82(967), 315-322. doi:10.1136/pgmj.2005.042200

Question 3.2

Which of the following statements about the relation between obesity and sleep apnea is correct?

a. Apnea-hypopnea index is likely to increase with an increase in BMI.

b. Apnea-hypopnea index is likely to decrease with an increase in BMI.

c. Apnea-hypopnea index is unlikely to decrease with a decrease in BMI.

d. Apnea-hypopnea index has an inverse relation with a change in BMI.

e. None of the above statements are correct.

The correct answer is "a."

Increasing BMI has a close association with the development of obstructive sleep apnea. It may also worsen the pre-existing condition. Apnea-hypopnea index is a ratio to determine the severity of sleep apnea.

Schmid, S. M., Hallschmid, M., & Schultes, B. (2015). The metabolic burden of sleep loss. The Lancet Diabetes & Endocrinology, 3(1), 52-62. doi:10.1016/s2213-8587(14)70012-9

Question 3.3

Obesity is known to have a paradoxical effect on which one of the following conditions?

   a. Diabetes type 2
   b. Essential hypertension
   c. Obstructive sleep apnea
   d. Congestive heart failure (CHF)
   e. Arthritis

The correct answer is "d."

Paradoxical effect on CHF is sometimes noted with obesity. It is observed that weight loss may worsen CHF in some cases.

Kenchaiah, S., Evans, J. C., Levy, D., Wilson, P. W., Benjamin, E. J., Larson, M. G., . . . Vasan, R. S. (2002). Obesity and the Risk of Heart Failure. New England Journal of Medicine, 347(5), 305-313. doi:10.1056/nejmoa020245

Question 3.4

Weight loss is unlikely to improve which of the following conditions?

    a. Diabetes type 2

    b. Obstructive sleep apnea

    c. Osteoporosis

    d. Risk of multi-organ cancer

    e. Fatty liver

The correct answer is "c."

All the conditions stated above are likely to improve with losing weight, except osteoporosis. It is risk remains unchanged in most cases.

Shapses, Sue A., and Deeptha Sukumar. Annual Review of Nutrition, U.S. National Library of Medicine, 21 Aug. 2012, www.ncbi.nlm.nih.gov/pmc/articles/PMC4016236/.

Question 3.5

Various cancers are more common in the obese population. The risk of which of the following cancer types does <u>not</u> increase with increasing BMI?

    a. Breast cancer

    b. Colon cancer

    c. Endometrial cancer

    d. Lung cancer

    e. Pancreas

The correct answer is "d."

All cancers stated above have increased risk in obese patients, except lung cancer.

Question 3.6

Adipose tissues are recognized for generating both pro-inflammatory and anti-inflammatory components. Which of the subsequent assertions could be applicable to an individual with obesity?

   a. Increased tumor necrosis factor-α and interlukin-6

   b. Decreased tumor necrosis factor-α, interleukin-6, leptin, and plasminogen activator inhibitor.

   c. Increased adiponectin, interleukin 4-10, and interlukin-1 receptor antagonist

   d. Decreased leptin and plasminogen activator inhibitor.

   e. Increased interleukin-1 receptor antagonist

The correct answer is "a."

In obese individuals, increased levels of inflammatory cytokines are seen. Tumor necrosis factor-α and interleukin-6 levels are increased.

Odegaard, J. I., & Chawla, A. (2013). Pleiotropic Actions of Insulin Resistance and Inflammation in Metabolic Homeostasis. Science, 339(6116), 172-177. doi:10.1126/science.1230721

Question 3.7

A link between diabetes and obesity is well established. Which of the following statements is <u>not</u> correct in this regard?

    a. Over 80% of individuals with diabetes are classified as obese, exhibiting android body morphology and elevated waist-to-hip ratios.

    b. Insulin resistance leads to more visceral fat accumulation.

    c. Even 5 to 10% weight loss can help bring glycemic control.

    d. Diabetic medications such as incretin mimetics (e.g., exenatide) are likely to cause weight loss.

    e. Sulfonylureas and thiazolidinediones are likely to cause weight loss.

The correct answer is "e."

Sulfonylureas (Amaryl®, Glucotrol®, diabeta®) and thiazolidinediones (Actos®, Avandia®) are known to cause potential weight gain. Statements "a." to "d." are correct.

Hevener, A. L., & Febbraio, M. A. (2010). The 2009 Stock Conference Report: Inflammation, Obesity, and Metabolic Disease. Obesity Reviews, 11(9), 635-644. doi:10.1111/j.1467-789x.2009.00691.x

*Amaryl® and diabeta® are registered trademarks of Sanofi-aventis U.S. LLC, Glucotrol® is a registered trademark of Pfizer Inc., Actos® is a registered trademark of Takeda Pharmaceutical Company, Avandia® is a registered trademark of GlaxoSmithKline plc.

Question 3.8

In terms of obesity and cardiovascular disease, which of the ensuing statements is accurate?

a. The risk of cardiovascular disease in obese, diabetic women and men is 78.8% and 86.9% respectively.

b. Patients with a high BMI who manifest congestive heart failure (CHF) experience a reduced risk of hospitalization and mortality compared to individuals with a normal BMI in similar circumstances.

c. Anorectic medications should be employed cautiously in individuals with substantial cardiovascular disease.

d. Weight gain resulting in an increase in BMI from below 25 to above 30 is correlated with a rise in the prevalence of hypertension (HTN) from 15% to 40%.

e. All the above statements are correct.

The correct answer is "e."

Statements "a." to "d." are all correct. This question discusses the high cardiovascular risks in obese patients. There seems to be the paradoxical effect of obesity on congestive heart failure.

Wilson, P. W., Dagostino, R. B., Sullivan, L., Parise, H., & Kannel, W. B. (2002). Overweight and Obesity as Determinants of Cardiovascular Risk. Archives of Internal Medicine, 162(16), 1867. doi:10.1001/archinte.162.16.1867

Question 3.9

Which of the following is not the component of diagnostic criteria for metabolic syndrome?

    a. Abdominal waist circumference

    b. Triglycerides and fasting blood sugar

    c. High-density lipoprotein

    d. Blood pressure

    e. Liver function tests

The correct answer is "e."

Liver function abnormality is not encompassed in the diagnostic criteria for metabolic syndrome, while all other facts mentioned in statements "a" to "d" are considered.

Phelan, S., Wadden, T. A., Berkowitz, R. I., Sarwer, D. B., Womble, L. G., Cato, R. K., & Rothman, R. (2007). Impact of weight loss on the metabolic syndrome. International Journal of Obesity, 31(9), 1442-1448. doi: 10.1038/sj.ijo.0803606

Question 3.10

Which of the following statements is <u>not</u> correct regarding the relation between obesity and renal disease?

a. Most common renal lesion seen in obese individuals is focal and segmental glomerulosclerosis and glomerulomegaly.

b. Excessive weight gain may lead to decreased renal tubular sodium reabsorption and compensatory renal vasoconstriction.

c. Proteinuria may develop in obese individuals due to nephron damage.

d. High waist circumference has an association with poor renal function.

The correct answer is "b."

All statements except "b." are correct. Weight gain leads to increased reabsorption of renal tubular sodium and compensatory renal vasodilation.

Burton, J. O., Gray, L. J., Webb, D. R., Davies, M. J., Khunti, K., Crasto, W., . . . Brunskill, N. J. (2011). Association of anthropometric obesity measures with chronic kidney disease risk in a non-diabetic patient population. Nephrology Dialysis Transplantation, 27(5), 1860-1866. doi:10.1093/ndt/gfr574

Question 3.11

Which of the following statements is correct about the estimated glomerular filtration rate (GFR) in patients after bariatric surgery?

   a. Estimated GFR remains one of the most reliable methods of renal function assessment.

   b. Estimated GFR does not depend on creatinine.

   c. Estimated GFR is likely to decrease in post-bariatric patients due to loss of muscle mass.

   d. Estimated GFR does not take into account the surface area of the patient.

   e. Estimated GFR may increase without real improvement of renal function.

The correct answer is "e."

This intriguing observation is based on multiple findings. Following bariatric surgery, patients experience a reduction in muscle mass. Additionally, the GFR data tables are derived from non-obese patients, and GFR calculations are not adjusted for decreased surface area after weight loss. This concern can potentially result in inaccurate GFR estimations. Several equations used in GFR assessment, such as CKD-EPI, MDRD, and Cockcroft-Gault, have been utilized, with the latter incorporating adjustments for lean body mass.

Editorial Board. (2016). Surgery for Obesity and Related Diseases, 12(1), I-li. doi:10.1016/s1550-7289(15)01029-1

Question 3.12

A 70-year-old patient undergoes gastric bypass surgery. His outcomes may differ from a 40-year-old who receives the same type of surgery. Which of the following statements is correct?

   a. He is likely to have more excess weight loss.
   b. His chances of having complications are less.
   c. He has better chances to have remission of sleep apnea.
   d. Type 2 diabetes remission chances are higher.
   e. "a." and "c." are correct.

The correct answer is "e."

The older age group has more chances of post-operative complications. Younger patients may see a remission of diabetes more often. However, the older age group sees more excess weight loss and has better resolution of sleep apnea.

Question 3.13

A morbidly obese patient undergoes a sleep study as part of the preoperative assessment for bariatric surgery. The sleep study report indicates six central apneas, 78 hypopneas, and an Apnea Hypopnea Index (AHI) of 17 per hour. The minimum oxygen saturation recorded was 85%. During his follow-up appointment with his family physician, the sleep study report was reviewed. Which of the subsequent statements is accurate concerning his findings?

   a. His AHI index is normal.
   b. His AHI index indicates mild sleep apnea.
   c. His AHI index suggests moderate sleep apnea.
   d. His AHI index suggests severe sleep apnea.
   e. AHI is not particularly important in the prediction of sleep apnea.

The correct answer is "c."

An Apnea Hypopnea Index (AHI) below 5 is considered normal, while a range of 5 to 15 is classified as mild. An AHI between 15 to 30 falls into the moderate category, and a value exceeding 30 is deemed severe. Recommendations for managing such cases include improving sleep hygiene, weight loss, employing positional therapy, avoiding alcohol and nicotine-containing products. Furthermore, it is advisable to undergo CPAP/BPAP titration to determine the optimal positive pressure level for therapeutic purposes. Sleep apnea can manifest as central or obstructive types.

In central apnea, there is a simultaneous halt in both oral and nasal airflow alongside the cessation of respiratory movements for a minimum duration of 10 seconds. In contrast, obstructive apnea is characterized by the cessation of airflow while respiratory movements persist.

Shamsuzzaman, Abu S. M., et al. "Obstructive Sleep Apnea." Jama, vol. 290, no. 14, Aug. 2003, p. 1906., doi:10.1001/jama.290.14.1906.

Question 3.14

What is a correct statement about the definition of hypopnea?

a. Decreased flow > 30% from baseline for 20 seconds.

b. Decreased flow > 30% from baseline for 10 seconds.

c. Decreased flow > 40% from baseline for 5 seconds.

d. Decreased flow > 50% from baseline for 10 seconds.

e. Decreased flow > 50% from baseline for 20 seconds.

The correct answer is "b."

Decreased flow > 30% from the baseline for 10 seconds is considered significant to confirm the diagnosis of a hypopnea event.

5th Edition Obesity – Relation with Other Diseases

Question 3.15

Morbid obesity has a close association with obstructive sleep apnea. Determining the Apnea-Hypopnea Index (AHI) is essential in assessing the magnitude of obstructive sleep apnea. Which of the following statements is correct regarding calculation of AHI?

a. AHI = (numbers of apneas + numbers of hypopneas) / sleep hours

b. AHI = sleep hours / (numbers of apneas + numbers of hypopneas)

c. AHI = (numbers of apneas - numbers of hypopneas) / sleep hours

d. AHI = sleep hours / (numbers of apneas - numbers of hypopneas)

e. AHI= (numbers of apneas + numbers of hypopneas + Respiratory Effort Related Arousal (RERAs) / sleep hours

The correct answer is "a."

AHI is determined by the sum of the numbers of apneas and number of hypopneas, divided by sleep hours.

The Apnea-Hypopnea Index (AHI) is computed by adding the count of apneas and hypopneas and then dividing this sum by the total sleep duration in hours. The AHI can be further divided into obstructive AHI and central AHI. Additionally, separate indices for Apnea (AI) and Hypopnea (HI) may be reported individually.

Among these measurements, the total AHI is the most commonly used to assess the severity of sleep apnea. For adults, an obstructive AHI exceeding 15 (or exceeding 5 in the presence of relevant signs, symptoms, or comorbidities) meets the diagnostic criteria for obstructive sleep apnea (OSA). To formally diagnose central sleep apnea (CSA), a central AHI of at least five events per hour is required.

Question 3.16

Untreated obstructive sleep apnea demonstrates a significant association with morbid obesity, potentially leading to a range of adverse outcomes. Without intervention, individuals afflicted by both morbid obesity and sleep apnea face an elevated susceptibility to which of the subsequent conditions?

   a. Congestive heart failure (CHF)
   b. Atrial fibrillation
   c. Cerebrovascular events
   d. Hypertension
   e. Pulmonary hypertension
   f. All above statements are correct.

The correct answer is "f."

Obesity and sleep apnea have a close association. Endothelial damage via various mechanisms and repeated hypoxia leads to the production of oxidative stress. It can lead to enhanced atherosclerosis potential through the production of inflammatory cytokines.

Question 3.17

Several medications are known to affect lipid and carbohydrate metabolism. Which of the following medications may lead to hyperglycemia, lipid disorder, decreased subcutaneous fat, and more visceral fat accumulation?

   a. Loop diuretics

   b. Proton pump inhibitors

   c. Antiretroviral therapy

   d. Cephalosporins

   e. Chronic coumadin use.

The correct answer is "c."

HIV-associated lipodystrophy" typically involves alterations in fat distribution accompanied by metabolic issues such as dyslipidemia and insulin resistance. It can manifest as lipoatrophy (loss of subcutaneous fat in limbs, face, or buttocks) or fat accumulation (visceral fat gain, buffalo hump, and breast enlargement). Treatment strategies vary based on the type of fat change, with lipoatrophy and fat accumulation. Antiretroviral therapy is noted to have stated side effects. The primary contributor to lipoatrophy is the use of thymidine analogues, particularly stavudine and zidovudine. Therefore, the primary medical strategy for addressing lipoatrophy involves changing the antiretroviral regimen by substituting stavudine or zidovudine with alternative NRTIs, such as tenofovir or abacavir. Metformin may help in preventing some of these effects.

Question 3.18

A 48-year-old woman is contemplating bariatric surgery to address her lifelong issue of morbid obesity. Additionally, she is currently dealing with perimenopausal symptoms and has been extensively researching them online. During her next appointment with her family physician, she raises several inquiries regarding osteoporosis and its potential implications for her age and weight loss surgery. The family physician provides detailed information about various facets of osteoporosis. Please choose the correct statement.

a. Weight loss with bariatric surgery will potentially cause her to lose bone mass density.

b. Bone loss is more pronounced in perimenopausal women and older men

c. Trabecular bones lose more density as compared to other sites.

d. Older individuals losing more than 10% of weight carry more risk of hip fracture.

e. All the above statements are correct.

The correct answer is "e."

Several studies have looked at the association of loss of bone density with weight loss. It potentially increases the risk of fractures in older individuals of both sexes. Hip and distal forearms are two common fracture sites in this group. Shapses, Sue A., and Deeptha Sukumar. Annual Review of Nutrition, U.S. National Library of Medicine, 21 Aug. 2012, www.ncbi.nlm.nih.gov/pmc/articles/PMC4016236/.

Question 3.19

A 39-year-old female with morbid obesity has abnormal liver functions for the last two years. She has a BMI of 53. Gastroenterology and bariatric consultations were requested. Liver biopsy was done at the time of bariatric surgery. The histopathology report revealed 40% macrovesicular steatosis. A follow up visit was arranged with her physician and the severity of steatosis was explained to her. Please select the correct statement.

a. She has severe hepatic steatosis.

b. She has moderate hepatic steatosis.

c. She has mild hepatic steatosis.

d. If ballooning degeneration is present, it is the characteristic sign of steatohepatitis.

e. "b" and "d" statements are correct.

The correct answer is "e."

On microscopic examination, less than 5% steatosis is considered normal. 5 to 33% is mild, 34 to 66% is moderate, and more than 66% is severe. Ballooning degeneration determines the presence of steatohepatitis.
"Nonalcoholic Steatohepatitis (NASH)." Pathology Outlines - PathologyOutlines.com,
www.pathologyoutlines.com/topic/liverNASH.html.

Question 3.20

Some sleep labs report Respiratory effort-related arousals (RERAs) in sleep study reports in addition to apnea hypopnea index (AHI). Which of the following statements about Respiratory effort-related arousals (RERAs) is accurate?

a. RERAs are formally defined as events lasting at least 5 seconds.
b. Scoring of RERAs is a mandatory requirement in the AASM scoring manual.
c. There is minimal interobserver variation in scoring RERAs compared to apneas and hypopneas.
d. Many laboratories report sleep-disordered breathing severity both with and without inclusion of RERAs.

The correct answer is "d."

Some sleep labs use the Respiratory Disturbance Index (RDI), calculated by adding apneas, hypopneas, and RERAs and dividing by total sleep hours. RDI, including RERAs, yields higher values than AHI but may have more scoring variability. Although RERAs might not consistently link to cardiovascular issues, they can negatively affect neurocognitive function. Thus, RDI provides unique clinical insights compared to AHI despite its limitations.

https://www.uptodate.com/contents/polysomnography-in-the-evaluation-of-sleep-disordered-breathing-in-adults?search=calculatin%20of%20apnea%20hypopnea%20index&source=search_result&selectedTitle=1~69&usage_type=default&display_rank=1

Question 3.21

A 50-year-old female with a BMI of 42 kg/m² and a history of severe obstructive sleep apnea (OSA) presents to the clinic for follow-up. She has been on continuous positive airway pressure (CPAP) therapy for the past six months. Despite this, she continues to experience daytime somnolence, fatigue, and morning headaches. Her spouce reports that she has frequent pauses in breathing during sleep. Her arterial blood gas (ABG) shows a pH of 7.35, PaCO2 of 52 mmHg, and bicarbonate of 29 mmol/L. Her serum bicarbonate level was previously measured at 28 mmol/L. Obesity hypoventilation syndrome (OHS) is suspected.

Lab Results:

Serum Bicarbonate: 28 mmol/L (normal range: 22-28 mmol/L)
Arterial Blood Gas: pH 7.35, PaCO2 52 mmHg, Bicarbonate 29 mmol/L (normal range for bicarbonate: 22-28 mmol/L)

Question:
   a. What is the most appropriate next step in the management of this patient?
   b. Increase the CPAP pressure settings
   c. Switch to noninvasive ventilation (NIV)
   d. Initiate weight-loss interventions, including bariatric surgery
   e. Measure arterial blood gases again in one month

The correct answer is "b."

Given the patient's symptoms and ABG results, which show elevated PaCO2 and bicarbonate levels, she likely has obesity hypoventilation syndrome (OHS) despite CPAP therapy. While increasing CPAP pressure might be beneficial in managing severe OSA, it is not sufficient for OHS. Switching to noninvasive ventilation (NIV) is recommended to ensure adequate ventilation and improve gas exchange in patients with OHS. Weight-loss interventions, including bariatric surgery, are crucial for long-term management but not the immediate next step. Repeating the ABG in one month is not immediately necessary if clinical suspicion of OHS is high.

Mokhlesi B, Masa JF, Brozek JL, Gurubhagavatula I, Murphy PB, Piper AJ, Tulaimat A, Afshar M, Balachandran JS, Dweik RA, Grunstein RR, Hart N, Kaw R, Lorenzi-Filho G, Pamidi S, Patel BK, Patil SP, Pépin JL, Soghier I, Tamae Kakazu M, Teodorescu M. Evaluation and Management of Obesity Hypoventilation Syndrome. An Official American Thoracic Society Clinical Practice Guideline. Am J Respir Crit Care Med. 2019 Aug 1;200(3):e6-e24. doi: 10.1164/rccm.201905-1071ST. Erratum in: Am J Respir Crit Care Med. 2019 Nov 15;200(10):1326. doi: 10.1164/rccm.v200erratum7. PMID: 31368798; PMCID: PMC6680300.

Question 3.22

Which of the following statements is true regarding Obesity Hypoventilation Syndrome (OHS)?

a. OHS is characterized by a BMI ≥ 35 kg/m², sleep-disordered breathing, and daytime hypercapnia (PaCO2 ≥ 55 mm Hg).
b. OHS is exclusively found in patients with obstructive sleep apnea (OSA) with an apnea-hypopnea index (AHI) ≥ 25 events per hour.
c. Positive airway pressure (PAP) therapy is the primary management option for controlling sleep-disordered breathing and reversing daytime hypoventilation in patients with OHS.
d. The prevalence of OHS is well-documented in the general population and is found to be around 50%.

The correct answer is "c."
Obesity Hypoventilation Syndrome (OHS) is characterized by obesity (BMI ≥ 30 kg/m²), sleep-disordered breathing (SDB), and awake daytime hypercapnia (PaCO2 ≥ 45 mm Hg), after excluding other hypoventilation causes. This condition is a severe form of obesity-related respiratory compromise, leading to increased mortality, chronic heart failure, pulmonary hypertension, and frequent hospitalizations for acute-on-chronic hypercapnic respiratory failure. The rising prevalence of severe obesity (BMI ≥ 40 kg/m²) worldwide has contributed to an increase in OHS cases, particularly among patients referred to sleep centers for SDB evaluation. Approximately 90% of OHS patients also have obstructive sleep apnea (OSA), necessitating polysomnography for accurate diagnosis. Positive airway pressure (PAP) therapy, including noninvasive ventilation (NIV) or continuous PAP (CPAP), is the primary treatment to manage SDB and reverse

hypoventilation in OHS patients. Despite available treatments, many OHS patients are not diagnosed until severe complications arise, underscoring the importance of early recognition and intervention to improve outcomes.
Balachandran JS, Masa JF, Mokhlesi B. Obesity hypoventilation syndrome epidemiology and diagnosis. Sleep Med Clin. 2014;9:341–347

Question 3.23

A 55-year-old woman visits her primary care physician for a routine check-up. She has a BMI of 30 kg/m², reports limited physical activity, and occasionally smokes. She consumes alcohol moderately and maintains a diet that she describes as "average." Her physician advises her on the benefits of adopting a healthier lifestyle, including quitting smoking, losing weight, increasing physical activity, moderating alcohol intake, and improving her diet quality. Which of the following statements best reflects the potential impact of adopting all five low-risk lifestyle factors on this patient's life expectancy and mortality risk?

a. Adopting all five low-risk lifestyle factors can increase life expectancy at age 50 by approximately 14 years for women compared to those with none of the low-risk factors.
b. Adopting all five low-risk lifestyle factors primarily reduces the risk of cancer mortality, with minimal impact on cardiovascular disease mortality.
c. The population-attributable risk of nonadherence to the five low-risk factors is approximately 30% for all-cause mortality.
d. The multivariable-adjusted hazard ratio for all-cause mortality in adults with five low-risk factors compared to those with none is 0.50.

The correct answer is "a."

A recent study indicated that adopting all five low-risk lifestyle factors significantly increases life expectancy and reduces mortality risk. Women who adopted all five factors had an estimated life expectancy at age 50 of 43.1 years, compared to 29.0 years for those with none of the low-risk factors, resulting in a difference of approximately 14 years. The study also showed substantial reductions in all-cause mortality, cancer mortality, and cardiovascular disease mortality for individuals with five low-risk factors compared to those with none.

Li Y, Pan A, Wang DD, et al. Impact of healthy lifestyle factors on life expectancies in the US population. Circulation. 2018;138(4):345-355. doi:10.1161/circulationaha.117.032047

Question 3.24

A 55-year-old female patient with a BMI of 33 kg/m² presents to your clinic for a routine check-up. She is concerned about her risk of developing obesity-related diseases. Her recent lab results show normal glucose levels, normal lipid profile, and no hypertension. She exercises regularly and reports no significant health issues. You discuss with her the concept of metabolically healthy obesity (MHO) and the potential risks and benefits associated with her condition. Which of the following statements is most accurate regarding the management of metabolically healthy obesity (MHO)?

a. Individuals with MHO have no increased risk of cardiovascular diseases compared to healthy lean individuals.
b. MHO is a stable condition that does not require therapeutic weight loss.
c. MHO individuals have lower amounts of ectopic fat and preserved insulin sensitivity compared to those with unhealthy obesity.
d. The absence of metabolic abnormalities in MHO eliminates the need for regular monitoring and lifestyle interventions.

The correct answer is "c."
Metabolically healthy obesity (MHO) is characterized by normal glucose and lipid metabolism and the absence of hypertension, despite the presence of obesity. Individuals with MHO typically have lower amounts of ectopic fat (such as visceral and liver fat) and higher leg fat deposition. They also exhibit better expandability of subcutaneous adipose tissue, preserved insulin sensitivity, and beta-cell function, as well as better cardiorespiratory fitness compared to those with unhealthy obesity. While MHO may confer a lower risk of cardiometabolic diseases compared to metabolically unhealthy obesity, the risk is still higher compared to healthy lean individuals. Additionally, MHO is often a transient state, and therapeutic weight loss may still be beneficial. Therefore, regular monitoring and

lifestyle interventions are important for managing MHO and reducing the risk of progression to unhealthy obesity.

Blüher M. Metabolically Healthy Obesity. Endocr Rev. 2020 May 1;41(3):bnaa004. doi: 10.1210/endrev/bnaa004. PMID: 32128581; PMCID: PMC7098708.

Question 3.25

A 50-year-old male with type 2 diabetes and a BMI of 31 kg/m² is concerned about the potential risks of cancer associated with his antidiabetic medications. He is currently taking metformin and his doctor is considering adding a second medication to better control his blood sugar levels. The patient is aware of various medications, including sulphonylureas, insulin, thiazolidinediones (TZDs), and incretin-based drugs, but he is worried about their possible cancer risks based on what he has read.

Which of the following statements is true regarding the association between antidiabetic medications and cancer risk?

a. Metformin is associated with a significant increase in cancer risk due to its direct tumorigenic properties.
b. Sulphonylureas have consistently been shown to reduce cancer risk in patients with type 2 diabetes.
c. Thiazolidinediones (TZDs) have been linked to an increased risk of bladder cancer.
d. Incretin-based drugs, such as GLP-1 receptor agonists, are confirmed to increase the risk of pancreatic cancer in human studies.

The correct answer is "c."

Metformin has been studied extensively for its potential impact on cancer risk. Early observational studies suggested that metformin might reduce cancer risk, but subsequent studies accounting for biases have shown null associations. There is strong biological evidence supporting metformin's antitumor effects, and ongoing clinical trials are evaluating its potential as an adjunct to cancer treatments.

The evidence regarding sulphonylureas and cancer risk is mixed, with some studies suggesting an increased risk, others showing no association, and a few even indicating a protective effect. This inconsistency is partly due to challenges in finding appropriate comparator groups and biases in study design.

Thiazolidinediones (TZDs), particularly pioglitazone, have been associated with a small but statistically significant increased risk of bladder cancer. This has led to warnings from the Food and Drug Administration and the removal of these drugs from the market in some countries due to concerns about heart failure and myocardial infarction risks.

Incretin-based drugs, including GLP-1 receptor agonists and DPP-4 inhibitors, initially raised concerns about pancreatic and medullary thyroid cancer risks. However, recent studies have not confirmed these associations in humans. There are still some concerns about the potential link between DPP-4 inhibitors and cholangiocarcinoma, which requires further investigation.
Lega IC, Lipscombe LL. Review: Diabetes, Obesity, and Cancer-Pathophysiology and Clinical Implications. Endocr Rev. 2020 Feb 1;41(1):bnz014. doi: 10.1210/endrev/bnz014. PMID: 31722374.

Question 3.26

A 45-year-old patient with obesity presents to the clinic with complaints of fatigue and difficulty managing blood glucose levels despite adhering to a prescribed diet and exercise regimen. Laboratory tests reveal elevated fasting blood glucose levels and increased markers of inflammation. The patient is concerned about the risk of developing type 2 diabetes mellitus (T2DM) and seeks advice on the underlying mechanisms that might be contributing to insulin resistance.

Which of the following best explains how obesity-related inflammation contributes to insulin resistance in skeletal muscle?

   a. Increased secretion of anti-inflammatory cytokines by adipose tissue
   b. Decreased influx of fatty acids from visceral adipose tissue to skeletal muscle
   c. Increased immune cell infiltration and proinflammatory activation in intermyocellular and perimuscular adipose tissue
   d. Enhanced glucose uptake by myocytes due to chronic inflammation

The correct answer is "c."

Obesity is associated with chronic inflammation, which significantly contributes to the development of insulin resistance and type 2 diabetes mellitus (T2DM). Under normal conditions, skeletal muscle is responsible for the majority of insulin-stimulated whole-body glucose disposal. Dysregulation of skeletal muscle metabolism, particularly due to inflammation, can thus strongly influence whole-body glucose homeostasis and insulin sensitivity.

In the context of obesity, increased immune cell infiltration and proinflammatory activation occur within the intermyocellular and perimuscular adipose tissue. These immune cells secrete proinflammatory molecules that can induce inflammation in myocytes. This inflammation adversely regulates myocyte metabolism and contributes to insulin resistance through paracrine effects. Additionally, an increased influx of fatty acids and inflammatory molecules from other tissues, particularly visceral adipose tissue, further induces muscle inflammation and negatively affects myocyte metabolism, exacerbating insulin resistance.

In contrast, options a. and b. are incorrect as they do not accurately describe the mechanisms by which obesity-related inflammation contributes to insulin resistance. Option d. is incorrect because chronic inflammation does not enhance glucose uptake by myocytes; rather, it impairs it.

Question 3.27

A 55-year-old male with type 2 diabetes presents to the clinic for routine follow-up. He has a BMI of 37 kg/m² and a family history of cardiovascular disease. He is concerned about his risk of stroke, given his diabetes and family history.

Based on recent research findings, which of the following statements accurately describes the association between BMI and stroke risk in patients with type 2 diabetes?

a. Higher BMI is associated with an increased risk of total, ischemic, and hemorrhagic stroke in patients with type 2 diabetes.
b. There is no significant association between BMI and stroke risk in patients with type 2 diabetes.
c. Higher BMI is associated with a decreased risk of total, ischemic, and hemorrhagic stroke in patients with type 2 diabetes.
d. Patients with type 2 diabetes and a BMI within the normal range (18.5–24.9 kg/m²) have the lowest risk of stroke.

The correct answer is "c."

Recent research findings suggest an inverse relationship between BMI and the risk of total, ischemic, and hemorrhagic stroke in patients with type 2 diabetes. A large retrospective study involving over 67,000 patients showed that those with higher BMI categories experienced a lower incidence of stroke events. This consistent, graded inverse association was observed across various subgroups and remained significant even after adjusting for multiple confounding factors.

Shen Y, Shi L, Nauman E, Katzmarzyk PT, Price-Haywood EG, Bazzano AN, Nigam S, Hu G. Association between Body Mass Index and Stroke Risk Among Patients with Type 2 Diabetes. J Clin Endocrinol Metab. 2020 Jan 1;105(1):96–105. doi: 10.1210/clinem/dgz032. PMID: 31529060; PMCID: PMC6936963.

Question 3.28

A 35-year-old male with a BMI of 28.5 kg/m² reports consistently sleeping less than 6.5 hours per night. He is interested in lifestyle changes to aid in weight management. Based on the findings of a randomized clinical trial, what impact could extending his sleep duration to 8.5 hours per night have on his energy intake and weight?

a. Increased sleep duration would likely lead to an increase in total energy expenditure and weight loss.
b. Extending sleep duration would likely decrease daily energy intake without significantly affecting total energy expenditure, resulting in weight loss.
c. There would be no significant change in energy intake or expenditure, but sleep extension would improve overall well-being.
d. Extending sleep duration would increase daily energy intake due to more time awake, potentially leading to weight gain.

The correct answer is "b."

A recent randomized clinical tria demonstrated that extending sleep duration by approximately 1.2 hours per night led to a significant reduction in daily energy intake (around 270 kcal/day) without a significant change in total energy expenditure. This reduction in energy intake, combined with unchanged energy expenditure, resulted in a negative energy balance and subsequent weight loss. This suggests that adequate sleep duration could be an effective component of weight management and obesity prevention strategies.

Tasali E, Wroblewski K, Kahn E, Kilkus J, Schoeller DA. Effect of Sleep Extension on Objectively Assessed Energy Intake Among Adults With Overweight in Real-life Settings: A Randomized Clinical Trial. *JAMA Intern Med.* 2022;182(4):365-374. doi:10.1001/jamainternmed.2021.8098

Psychology and Counseling Aspects

Question 4.1

Motivational interview (MI) is a crucial component of managing behavioral modification in patients suffering from obesity. Which of the following statements is not correct about the motivational interview?

   a. It is a client-centered counseling style to elicit behavior change by clients to help explore and resolve ambivalence.

   b. MI can result in more weight loss and better maintenance.

   c. Collaboration rather than confrontation is a key component of MI.

   d. Close-ended questions can easily discover the patient's participation, goals, and values.

   e. Clinician provides resources to the patients to bring change.

   f. Generating gap to highlight discrepancy in goal setting, and roll with resistance are essential aspects of the motivational interview.

The correct answer is "d."

Close-ended questions are not particularly useful in determining a patient's goals, values, and health beliefs. All other statements are true. Client-centered counseling, motivational interview, collaboration, provision of resources to patients to bring changes, and to generate gap to express discrepancy are effective strategies.

Roberts, R. E., Deleger, S., Strawbridge, W. J., & Kaplan, G. A. (2003). Prospective association between obesity and depression: evidence from the Alameda County Study. International Journal of Obesity, 27(4), 514-521. doi: 10.1038/sj.ijo.0802204

Question 4.2

Several different psychological approaches and therapies are available for patients seeking help with the problem of obesity. Which of the following statements is true?

   a. Interpersonal therapy is an individualized approach with a focus to address emotional triggers and avoid relapsing into past habits.

   b. High prevalence of depression in obese patients requires screening on initial exam.

   c. Behavioral therapy has components involving positive and negative reinforcements.

   d. Cognitive therapy involves techniques to change ineffective thinking.

   e. Cognitive behavior therapy involves changes in cognitive understanding to enable the client to recognize various triggers which lead to self-defeating actions or behaviors

   f. All the above statements are correct

The correct answer is "f."

Interpersonal, behavioral, cognitive, and cognitive behavior therapies are essential elements of psychological interventions. A high percentage of bariatric cases have depression. This issue needs to be assessed at the initial examination.

Perri, M. G. (2014). Effects of behavioral treatment on long-term weight loss: Lessons learned from the look AHEAD trial. Obesity, 22(1), 3-4. doi:10.1002/oby.20672

Question 4.3

Motivational interview (MI) involves several stages. Please select the statement stating correct order.

    a. Action, preparation, contemplation, pre-contemplation, and relapse

    b. Action, contemplation, preparation, pre-contemplation, and relapse

    c. Contemplation, pre-contemplation, preparation, action, and relapse

    d. Preparation, action, pre-contemplation, contemplation, and relapse

    e. Pre-contemplation, contemplation, preparation, action, and relapse

The correct answer is "e."

Question 4.4

Motivational interview (MI) involves several components. A therapist uses a technique which can have variants including reflection, shifting focus, reframing, and siding with resistance. Please select the statement stating the type of technique described here.

   a. Roll with resistance.
   b. Therapeutic paradox
   c. Evocation
   d. Collaboration
   e. Pre-contemplation

The correct answer is "a."

Question 4.5

A 33-year-old female follows a bariatric practice. She weighs 325 lbs. She lives with her boyfriend and has several family stressors. She has six visits to the office in the last 14 months. At the start of the program, her weight was 324 lbs. She had a few appointments with the nutritionist too. Several medications to help her lose weight were tried at various times. The list of drugs includes phentermine, topiramate, and bupropion/naltrexone combination. She admits having several, poor eating habits. She likes cheese with crackers and consumes a large amount daily; it seems she is not willing to give up this habit. Her case was discussed in the multidisciplinary meeting of the practice and during her next visit, the counsellor tells her, "You have followed our program for a good amount of time. It looks as if you have too much going on in your life and it is not letting you make a change. I am wondering what our strategy could be going forward." Please select the statement which reflects the technique that the counsellor used on her to address the issue.

   a. Roll with resistance.
   b. Therapeutic paradox
   c. Evocation
   d. Collaboration
   e. Pre-contemplation

The correct answer is "b."

It is an example of a therapeutic paradox. The counselor comments and hopes that the patient may bring a thought or initiative to change the situation.

Question 4.6

A 37-year-old female joins a bariatric program. She is recently diagnosed with insulin resistance and impaired glucose tolerance. Her mother and one of the older sisters have diabetes. She is very scared of developing this disease. She makes a lot of dietary changes and goes to the gym regularly. She lost 20 labs in three months. At her follow-up visit her doctor is pleased with her progress. He says "You have done very well. Can you tell what changes in diet and lifestyle helped you to lose this much of weight"?

Please select the technique reflected by his statement.

a. Roll with resistance.
b. Therapeutic paradox
c. Affirmation
d. Collaboration
e. Pre-contemplation

The correct answer is "c."

It is an example of affirmation. These statements need to be real and relevant. The provider here recognizes the patient's strengths and effort to make a favorable change.

Question 4.7

Which principle of Motivational Interviewing (MI) emphasizes the importance of understanding and accepting a client's perspective without judgment, using techniques like active listening and reflective listening?

   a. Develop Discrepancy
   b. Avoid Argument
   c. Roll With Resistance
   d. Express Empathy

The correct answer is "d."

Express Empathy: MI centers around empathy, which means understanding and accepting another's perspective and feelings without judgment. Neutrality is crucial, as it doesn't imply approval or agreement. Active listening, reflective listening, and forming reflections are techniques used to convey empathy in MI.

Develop Discrepancy: MI differs from purely client-centered approaches by being directive. It aims to highlight the gap between a person's current situation and their desired state, helping them overcome ambivalence and motivating change. By emphasizing the disparity between present behavior and important goals or values, the counselor assists the client in recognizing the significance of change.

Avoid Argument: In MI, arguing for change with a client often triggers resistance. Instead of confronting resistance, MI counselors "roll" with it, meaning they avoid direct confrontation and seek alternative approaches when faced with client resistance. Resistance is seen as an opportunity to understand the client's perspective better and respond in a non-confrontational manner.

Roll With Resistance: Resistance is viewed as a signal that the client perceives the situation differently, rather than mere defiance. MI encourages clinicians to adapt to resistance by changing direction, listening more attentively, and maintaining a nonjudgmental and respectful attitude. Avoiding evoking resistance whenever possible and redirecting the client's energy toward positive change is emphasized.

Recognizing resistance involves observing common client behaviors that indicate resistance to treatment. MI provides guidelines on how to respond appropriately to client resistance, with various strategies aimed at maintaining a non-confrontational and empathetic approach.

These principles collectively form the foundation of Motivational Interviewing, a counseling approach aimed at helping individuals overcome ambivalence and enhance their motivation for positive change.

Motivational Interviewing 101 - A Short Guide to Understanding MI By Stephen L. Reese, MPA, MS and Lamont Clark, MBA.

Question 4.8

Which treatment is recommended as the first-line approach for binge eating disorder?

   a. Interpersonal psychotherapy
   b. Medication therapy
   c. Cognitive-Behavioral Therapy (CBT)
   d. Nutritional counseling

The correct answer is "c."

What percentage of patients who received therapist-led CBT achieved abstinence from binge eating episodes?

   a. 20%
   b. 59%
   c. 35%
   d. 11%

The correct answer is "b."

Question 4.9

What is the significance of a rapid response in the context of CBT treatment for binge eating disorder?

    a. It indicates a higher risk of treatment failure.
    b. It suggests a need for medication intervention.
    c. It is associated with higher rates of remission.
    d. It prolongs the duration of treatment.

The correct answer is "c."

Question 4.10

In which setting is self-help CBT for binge eating disorder potentially less effective?

    a. Primary care clinics
    b. Specialty eating disorder clinics.
    c. Outpatient psychotherapy centers
    d. Inpatient hospital settings

The correct answer is "a."

Question 4.11

What is a notable feature of self-help CBT tailored to binge eating disorder?

    a. It primarily focuses on obesity management.
    b. It is less effective than nonspecific self-help approaches.
    c. It often results in rapid remission.
    d. It can be as effective as therapist-led CBT and maintains improvement over time.

The correct answer is "d."

Cognitive-Behavioral Therapy (CBT) is the recommended first-line treatment for binge eating disorder. It is widely studied and considered the primary approach. CBT can be therapist-led for individuals or groups, or delivered through self-help programs. Studies show CBT's efficacy, with rapid symptom reduction signaling positive outcomes. However, patients with a history of anorexia or bulimia may have poorer results. Self-help CBT is also effective, particularly in specialty settings, and tailored self-help approaches work best. These interventions lead to sustained improvement and are often as effective as therapist-led CBT.

5th Edition Psychology and Counseling Aspects

Question 4.12

A 56-year-old patient with obesity is interested in participating in a weight loss program. Her healthcare provider mentions the Centers for Medicare and Medicaid Services (CMS) initiated coverage of intensive behavioral therapy (IBT) for obesity. Based on recent research, what outcomes can the patient expect from the IBT protocol provided by CMS?

a. Immediate weight loss of 10% within the first month
b. An average weight loss of 5.4% of initial weight at 24 weeks and 6.1% at 1 year
c. No significant weight loss but improved cardiovascular health
d. Complete resolution of obesity within 6 months

The correct answer is "d."

The research on the CMS IBT protocol showed that participants lost a mean of 5.4% of their initial weight at 24 weeks, with 46% of participants losing greater than or equal to 5% of their baseline weight. At 1 year, the mean weight loss was 6.1%, with 44% of participants achieving a weight loss of 5% or more. These results indicate modest but significant weight loss over time with the IBT protocol.

Centers for Medicare and Medicaid Services (CMS). (2023). Intensive behavioral therapy (IBT) for obesity: Review of evidence and protocol development. Pediatrics, 151(2), e2022060640.

A 45-year-old female patient with a BMI of 38.9 kg/m^2 is struggling to lose weight and maintain weight loss. She is considering joining a commercial weight management program and wants to know which strategies are effective for long-term weight maintenance.

Question 4.13

Which of the following strategies are commonly used by individuals who successfully maintain significant weight loss?

   a. Engaging in less frequent healthy dietary choices and self-monitoring.

   b. Ignoring food cravings and having greater habit strength for healthy eating.

   c. Practicing more frequent psychological coping strategies but less self-monitoring.

   d. Having a lower willingness to ignore food cravings and practicing fewer healthy dietary choices.

The correct answer is "b."

Successful weight loss maintainers often practice more frequent healthy dietary choices, self-monitoring, and psychological coping strategies. They also show a greater willingness to ignore food cravings and have stronger habits for healthy eating compared to those who do not maintain weight loss.

Phelan S, Halfman T, Pinto AM, Foster GD. Behavioral and Psychological Strategies of Long-Term Weight Loss Maintainers in a Widely Available Weight Management Program. Obesity (Silver Spring). 2020 Feb;28(2):421-428. doi: 10.1002/oby.22685. PMID: 31970912; PMCID: PMC7003766.

Question 4.14

A 50-year-old female with a BMI of 36 kg/m² presents to a primary care clinic that serves a predominantly low-income population. She has a history of hypertension and prediabetes. The clinic participates in a cluster-randomized trial aimed at evaluating the effectiveness of a high-intensity, lifestyle-based obesity treatment program delivered by health coaches embedded in the clinic. The program includes weekly sessions for the first 6 months, followed by monthly sessions for the next 18 months. Patients in the usual-care group receive standard care from their primary care team.

Which of the following outcomes is most likely to be observed in patients participating in the high-intensity lifestyle intervention compared to those receiving usual care after 24 months?

a. No significant difference in weight loss between the two groups.
b. Greater weight loss in the high-intensity lifestyle intervention group with a mean difference of -4.51 percentage points.
c. Higher incidence of serious adverse events in the high-intensity lifestyle intervention group.
d. Significant increase in BMI in the usual-care group compared to baseline.

The correct answer is "b."

In a cluster-randomized trial involving primary care clinics serving predominantly low-income populations, patients who participated in a high-intensity, lifestyle-based obesity treatment program experienced significantly greater weight loss at 24 months compared to those receiving usual care. The study showed a mean weight loss difference of -4.51 percentage points between the intervention and usual-care groups. There were no significant between-group differences in serious adverse events, making the high-intensity lifestyle intervention both effective and safe.

Katzmarzyk PT, Martin CK, Newton RL Jr, Apolzan JW, Arnold CL, Davis TC, Price-Haywood EG, Denstel KD, Mire EF, Thethi TK, Brantley PJ, Johnson WD, Fonseca V, Gugel J, Kennedy KB, Lavie CJ, Sarpong DF, Springgate B. Weight Loss in Underserved Patients - A Cluster-Randomized Trial. N Engl J Med. 2020 Sep 3;383(10):909-918. doi: 10.1056/NEJMoa2007448. PMID: 32877581; PMCID: PMC7493523.

Question 4.15

A 45-year-old female with a BMI of 35 kg/m² is enrolled in a behavioral weight loss intervention program aimed at reducing weight through lifestyle changes. The program focuses on reducing caloric intake and increasing physical activity. The patient expresses concerns about weight-related self-stigma, particularly feelings of self-devaluation and fear of stigma from others. Throughout the program, the patient's self-devaluation decreases, and she begins to adopt more weight control strategies.

Which of the following outcomes is most likely to be observed in this patient as a result of decreased self-devaluation during the weight loss intervention program?

a. Increased fear of enacted stigma and no significant change in weight loss.
b. No change in the use of weight control strategies and minimal weight loss.
c. Increased use of weight control strategies, leading to significant weight loss.
d. Increased self-devaluation and greater difficulty in achieving weight loss.

The correct answer is "c."

Decreases in self-devaluation during a behavioral weight loss intervention are associated with improved weight loss outcomes. This relationship is mediated by the increased use of weight control strategies. As the patient's self-devaluation decreases, they are more likely to engage in weight control behaviors, which contributes to more effective weight loss. The findings emphasize the importance of addressing self-

stigma in weight loss programs to enhance adherence to weight control strategies and improve overall outcomes.
Lillis J, Thomas JG, Olson K, Wing RR. Weight self-stigma and weight loss during behavioural weight loss intervention. Obes Sci Pract. 2019 Jan 11;5(1):21-27. doi: 10.1002/osp4.314. PMID: 30847224; PMCID: PMC6381303.

Investigations for an Obese Patient

Question 5.1

A primary care physician encounters a morbidly obese patient in their office. Following a comprehensive history-taking session, a physical examination is conducted. The physician observes skin alterations characterized by pigmentation and maculopapular lesions, leading to a suspicion of acanthosis nigricans. Which of the following statements accurately describes this condition?

   a. It is likely to be present on the face, the front of neck and chest.

   b. HbA1c and glucose tolerance tests with fasting insulin levels should be done as part of the workup

   c. The color of rash is likely red to blue.

   d. Rash is unlikely to be present on the side or back of neck, axillae, or groins.

   e. None of the above statements are correct.

The correct answer is "b."

The usual distribution of this dark and blackish pigmentation is at the back of neck, axillae, and groins. Prevalence of diabetes is high in this group of patients, thus blood glucose and HbA1c need to be checked.

Hermanns-L T., Scheen, A., & Pierard, G. E. (2004). Acanthosis Nigricans Associated with Insulin Resistance. American Journal of Clinical Dermatology, 5(3), 199-203. doi:10.2165/00128071-200405030-00008

Investigations for an Obese Patient

Question 5.2

On further examination, the physician notices that the patient has a large abdominal pannus. This pannus extends to cover the upper thighs. What grade will be assigned to this pannus while documenting it in findings?

   a. Grade 1
   b. Grade 2
   c. Grade 3
   d. Grade 4
   e. Grade 5

The correct answer is "c."

A pannus extending to upper thighs is considered Grade 3. Other grades are as follows:

Grade 1 covers pubic hair; Grade 2 cover mons pubis; Grade 3 as stated above; Grade 4 extends to mid thighs; Grade 5 reaches the knees and beyond.

Panniculectomy Plastic Surgery Operation. (n.d.). Retrieved January 01, 2018, from http://www.bariatric-surgery.info/panniculectomy-surgical-procedure.htm

Investigations for an Obese Patient

Question 5.3

The physician measures the blood pressure of the patient after selecting an appropriate size cuff. Which of the following statements is correct regarding blood pressure measurement of a morbidly obese patient?

   a. The cuff should wrap less than one-third of the middle of the upper arm.

   b. The width of the cuff should not exceed arm diameter by 5%.

   c. The cuff should not wrap around two-thirds of the middle of the upper arm.

   d. Accurate reading cannot be taken with any blood pressure cuff.

   e. The width of the cuff should exceed diameter by 20%

The correct answer is "e."

The blood pressure readings may be falsely high if a smaller cuff is used for an obese patient. It is recommended that the bladder of the cuff should wrap around more than two-thirds of the middle of the upper arm and the width of the cuff should exceed 20 % of the diameter at the point of application. Upper arm circumference greater than 34 cm can be used as an indication to select a larger cuff size. For pediatric patients, it is recommended that the patient should be sitting for at least 5 minutes before the reading is taken and their feet should be kept on the ground. The bladder of the cuff should cover more than 80% of the circumference of mid-arm. The width of the cuff should exceed mid-arm circumference by 40%.

Investigations for an Obese Patient

Question 5.4

Regarding waist measurements, which of the following statements is correct?

a. The waist-hip circumference ratio of 0.7 in a male is a sign of central obesity.

b. The waist is measured at the level of the iliac crest, while the patient is standing and at the end of expiration.

c. The waist is measured while the patient is laying down with a deep breath in.

d. The tape around the waist should be adequately snug around the skin with good compression.

e. A waist to hip ratio of 1.2 defines it to be a gynecoid type of obesity with a strong association with metabolic syndrome.

The correct answer is "b."

The point of measurement is just above hip bones, it should not be compressing the skin and should be placed horizontally. In American males, waist circumference of 40 inches (102 cm) or above and females 35 inches (88 cm) or above is considered as the cut-off for abdominal obesity. It should be noted that BMI correlates better with metabolic disease as compared to waist circumference in patients with BMI ≥ 35kg/m². Cutoffs may be different for different racial and ethnic backgrounds.

Waist circumference of above 37 inches (94 cm) in middle aged males is a risk factor for development of type 2 diabetes and cardiovascular disease.

Assessing Your Weight. (2015, May 15). Retrieved December 28, 2017, from https://www.cdc.gov/healthyweight/assessing/Jacobson, Terry A., et al. "National Lipid Association Recommendations for Patient-Centered Management of Dyslipidemia: Part 1 – Executive Summary." Journal of Clinical Lipidology, vol. 8, no. 5, 2014, pp. 473–488., doi:10.1016/j.jacl.2014.07.007.

Question 5.5

Bioelectrical impedance (BIA) is commonly used in the workup of obese patients. Which of the following statements is correct regarding BIA?

   a. It has an advantage as it is not affected by the state of hydration.

   b. Fasting and recent exercise can alter BIA values.

   c. Fat mass has low impedance to flow of electric current.

   d. BIA has the advantage of being useful in extreme age groups.

   e. Low dose x-rays are used to measure the composition of body tissues.

The correct answer is "b."

Bioelectrical impedance (BIA) is an estimate of body fat mass and fat-free mass. Fat of the body and other tissues differ in characteristics of electrical impedance. BIA is rapid, easy to use and has virtually no safety concerns. Fasting, old age, hydration status and exercise may affect the value of BIA.

Bioelectric impedance analysis (BIA) is a widely used method for measuring body composition, although it has limitations. It involves measuring impedance, which is affected by electrode placement and body characteristics. Various formulas exist to convert impedance into estimates of fat content, but they often underestimate body fat. Accurate electrode placement and validated formulas are crucial for precise results. Recent advancements in BIA technology aim to improve accuracy by incorporating multiple frequencies and targeting multiple body segments.

Question 5.6

Which imaging technique is commonly used to determine patterns of body fat distribution, particularly by obtaining a single cross-sectional image at the interspace between the fourth and fifth lumbar vertebrae?

a. Positron emission tomography (PET)
b. Computed tomography (CT)
c. X-ray
d. Ultrasound

The correct answer is "b."

Imaging techniques play a vital role in assessing body fat distribution, with computed tomography (CT) and magnetic resonance imaging (MRI) being reliable methods. Typically, a single cross-sectional image at the fourth and fifth lumbar vertebrae is obtained to analyze subcutaneous and visceral fat. CT utilizes radiograph and computer analysis, offering high accuracy with minimal radiation exposure. On the other hand, MRI, which employs a powerful magnet, provides detailed images without radiation but requires longer scanning time. Nuclear magnetic resonance (NMR) spectroscopy, akin to MRI, distinguishes fat and glycogen within tissues. Although estimates of fat may vary among these methods, the relative ranking of subjects remains consistent.

Investigations for an Obese Patient

Question 5.7

Which of the following statements is not correct about "Brown Adipose Tissue"?

   a. Brown adipose tissue estimation can be done with PET scan.

   b. Lean individuals have more brown adipose content than obese individuals.

   c. Three-fourths of brown adipose content is found in cervical, supraclavicular, and axillary areas.

   d. Brown adipose tissue may have a key role in energy expenditure.

   e. Obese individuals carry more brown adipose tissue.

The correct answer is "e."

White adipose tissue (WAT) stores lipids, while brown adipose tissue (BAT) uses lipids for thermogenesis. Obesity leads to changes in WAT, causing expansion, dysfunction, and mild inflammation. Obese individuals typically have reduced BAT quantity and activity, primarily due to brown adipocyte conversion into white-like cells. Various factors, such as high temperature, leptin receptor deficiency, impaired β-adrenergic signaling, and lipase deficiency, trigger BAT "whitening," characterized by macrophage infiltration, brown adipocyte death, and crown-like structure formation.

Steelman, G. M., & Westman, E. C. Evaluation of the obese patient. In: Steelman, G. M., & Westman, E. C. (Eds.) Obesity:

evaluation and treatment essentials, 2nd Edition. Boca Raton: CRC Press, Taylor & Francis Group Press; 2016, pp.77-79

https://www.ncbi.nlm.nih.gov/pmc/articles/PMC5928436/#:~:text=In%20mammals%2C%20white%20adipose%20tissue,a%20low%2Dgrade%20inflammatory%20state.

Question 5.8

A 32-year-old woman visited her family doctor's office where her body composition was assessed using a body fat analyzer, revealing a fat percentage of 27%. Which of the following statements is accurate?

   a. She is likely to be an athlete.

   b. She should be regarded as obese.

   c. Her body fat percentage is not within an acceptable range.

   d. In women, 25 % of body fat is labeled as essential fat.

   e. If she loses 5% of her body fat, she would be in fitness range.

The correct answer is "e."

According to the American Council on Exercise classification, women with more than 32% body fat are considered obese, while levels between 25% to 31% are deemed acceptable. Fitness levels typically range between 21% to 24% body fat, while athletes usually have 14% to 20% body fat. For men, athletes typically have 6% to 13% body fat, fitness levels range from 14% to 17%, acceptable levels are between 18% to 24%, and obesity is classified as having more than 25% body fat.

Author Natalie Digate Muth Health and Fitness Expert Natalie Digate Muth. "What Are the Guidelines for Percentage of Body Fat Loss?" Body Fat Loss | Guidelines for Percentage of Body Fat Loss | ACE Blog, www.acefitness.org/education-and-resources/lifestyle/blog/112/what-are-the-guidelines-for-percentage-of-body-fat-loss.*

Question 5.9

A 28-year-old professional football player visits his primary care physician's office. He engages in vigorous exercise regularly. Standing at 5'11" tall, he weighs 260 lbs. Please choose the correct statement.

   a. Waist circumference will be more reliable in accessing adiposity.

   b. BMI measurement would give an appropriate assessment about his body fat.

   c. Body fat percentage calculation will be a better measure to assess body composition.

   d. None of the above statements is true.

The correct answer is "c."

In cases of exceptionally high muscle mass, such as in bodybuilders or individuals with sarcopenia, determining body fat percentage offers a more precise means of assessing body composition.

Question 5.10

In the evaluation of a bariatric patient, several tools are used. Which of the following is not an evaluation tool for sleep apnea?

a. Berlin Questionnaire

b. Stop-Bang Questionnaire

c. Epworth Scale

d. PHQ-9 Screen

The correct answer is "d."

The STOP-Bang questionnaire is widely acknowledged as the most validated tool for preoperative screening of obstructive sleep apnea (OSA). It comprises eight yes-or-no questions covering snoring, tiredness, observed apneas, among other factors, to categorize patients into low, intermediate, or high risk groups based on their total score. Research indicates a positive correlation between a higher STOP-Bang score and an increased likelihood of moderate to severe OSA. Moreover, combining elevated serum bicarbonate levels with an intermediate STOP-Bang score can improve specificity for predicting OSA. However, since not all factors in the questionnaire carry equal predictive value, a two-step scoring system has been proposed for intermediate-risk patients, involving a closer examination of specific items within the STOP criteria to enhance risk assessment. Additionally, different BMI thresholds may be warranted for various populations. Lastly, an intermediate to high-risk STOP-Bang score may signify an elevated risk of postoperative pulmonary and cardiac complications.

The Berlin questionnaire evaluates patients' risk for obstructive sleep apnea (OSA) by analyzing factors such as snoring, daytime sleepiness, hypertension, and BMI. It demonstrates a sensitivity of 69% for detecting OSA and 87% for severe OSA, but its specificity is moderate. Additionally, a Berlin score of ≥2 (indicating high risk) did not show a notable association with postoperative complications, ICU admission, or mortality in cohort studies, despite the data quality being evaluated as very low.

The Epworth Sleepiness Scale (ESS) assesses subjective sleepiness in everyday situations through eight scenarios, each rated from 0 to 3 based on dozing likelihood. Total scores range from 0 to 24, with higher values indicating more significant sleepiness. A score above 10 indicates excessive sleepiness, as found in observational studies. The ESS is easy to administer and adaptable to different settings. It moderately correlates with objective sleep measures and can track changes over time with repeated use.

PHQ- 9 (Patient Health Questionnaire) is used to screen depression. Options "a., "b." and "c." are used to assess sleep apnea. Stop-Bang Scale looks at some of the symptoms like snoring, tiredness, observed sleep apnea, blood pressure, age, circumference of the neck, and gender.

Biological Plausibility Linking Sleep Apnea and Metabolic ... https://www.nature.com/articles/nrendo.2016.22

"PHQ-9 Depression Test Questionnaire." Patient.info, Patient.info, patient.info/doctor/patient-health-questionnaire-phq-9.

https://www.uptodate.com/contents/surgical-risk-and-the-preoperative-evaluation-and-management-of-adults-with-obstructive-sleep-apnea?search=stop%20bang%20questionnaire&source=search_result&selectedTitle=1~16&usage_type=default&display_rank=1

https://www.uptodate.com/contents/quantifying-sleepiness?search=epworth%20sleepiness%20scale&source=search_result&selectedTitle=1~36&usage_type=default&display_rank=1

Question 5.11

Which of the following studies lacks utility in assessing the body composition of a morbidly obese patient?

a. Dual-energy X-ray absorptiometry
b. Bioelectric impedance
c. Near infrared interactance
d. QMR (quantitative magnetic resonance imaging)
e. Whole body air displacement plethysmography (BODPOD)
f. HIDA scan with CCK

The correct answer is "f."

HIDA scan with CCK is used to assess biliary and gallbladder function. All other items in statements "a." to "e." can be used to determine body fat composition.

Investigations for an Obese Patient

Question 5.12

When assessing an obese patient, it can be beneficial to determine both fat-free mass and lean body mass. Please choose the correct statement.

a. Lean body mass is total body mass minus fatty tissues. In a nonobese person it is generally 75% of total body mass

b. Fat-free mass is total body mass minus total body fat.

c. Lean body mass differs from the fat free mass by approximately 5%

d. Fat-free mass can be measured with techniques like dual-energy X-ray absorptiometry (DXA) scan or bioelectrical impedance (BIA)

e. All the above statements are correct

The correct answer is "e."

Fat-free mass comprises water, minerals, protein, and glycogen in the body. Conversely, lean body mass encompasses water, minerals, protein, glycogen, as well as the fat present in organs, bone marrow, and the central nervous system (CNS).

5th Edition Investigations for an Obese Patient

Question 5.13

A 65-year-old woman who underwent gastric bypass surgery 15 years ago has lost approximately 90 lbs. post-surgery. She was less compliant with follow-up care. She has regained a significant amount of weight over the years. During evaluation, various tests were conducted, including several scans, one of which provided T and Z scores. Upon reviewing her reports at the online portal for her records, she has questions about these scores at her follow-up visit. Please select the accurate statement.

 a. T and Z scores determine cardiovascular risk.

 b. T and Z scores determine diabetes development risk

 c. T and Z scores determine depression development risk

 d. T and Z scores determine osteoporosis development risk

 e. T and Z scores determine renal failure development risk

The correct answer is "d."

T and Z scores determine risk for osteoporosis. DXA scans can be used to identify this risk. Patients who are post-bariatric surgery, especially those who have gastric bypass, have a significant risk of osteoporosis. A T-score in range of -1 to -2.5 is regarded as osteopenia, and a score of -2.5 or below reflects osteoporosis. Normal level is -1 and above.

T-score compares the bone density of an individual with a 30-year-old healthy person of the same gender whereas Z score compares bone density with an average person of same gender and age.

Question 5.14

Measurements of basal and resting energy expenditure may provide useful insights into the management of obese patients. Please select the correct statement regarding calorimetry.

   a. Indirect calorimetry is done while the patient is in a chamber and measures the difference of the temperature of water entering and exiting the chamber
   b. Direct calorimetry estimates the energy expenditure by estimating consumption and production of oxygen and carbon dioxide respectively
   c. Respiratory quotient (RQ) = O_2consumed/CO_2 produced
   d. An RQ of 1.4 means lipolysis with underfeeding
   e. RQ of fats is 0.7

The correct answer is "e."

Indirect calorimetry is done with measurements of carbon dioxide produced and oxygen consumed. RQ for carbs and fats is 1 and 0.7, respectively. Low RQ is seen in ketosis. Its value is high in conditions of overfeeding and lipogenesis. RQ value below 0.85 reflects underfeeding. Respiratory Quotient (RQ) = CO_2 produced/O_2 consumed.

Sabounchi, N S, et al. "Best-Fitting Prediction Equations for Basal Metabolic Rate: Informing Obesity Interventions in Diverse Populations." International Journal of Obesity, vol. 37, no. 10, 2013, pp. 1364–1370., doi:10.1038/ijo.2012.218.

Question 5.15

Morbid obesity adversely affects the dynamics of breathing. Please select the correct statement.

a. Respiratory compliance is increased
b. Work of breathing is decreased
c. Functional residual capacity is increased
d. Closing volume to functional vital capacity ratio is high
e. Closing volume to functional vital capacity ratio is low

Correct answer is "e. "

In morbid obesity the respiratory compliance is decreased. The primary contributing factor is chest wall compliance. Recumbent position also adversely affects the condition. Work of breathing is increased with a decrease of functional residual capacity. Low ratio for closing volume explains the predisposition to atelectasis. This becomes clinically relevant in post-operative settings.

Question 5.16

Morbid obesity alters several respiratory dynamics and pulmonary function values. Please select the correct statement.

    a. FEV1 is likely to be high in an obese individual
    b. FEV1 is likely to be low in an obese patient
    c. FEV1 is likely to be the same for normal and morbidly obese individuals.
    d. In obese individuals, relationship between respiratory resistance and functional residual capacity (FRC) is linear

Correct answer is "b."

FEV1 is likely to be low in obese individuals and an inverse relationship exists between respiratory resistance and FRC.

https://www.scribd.com/document/618204555/Altered-Respiratory-Physiology-in-Obesity

Question 5.17

A super morbidly obese patient is seen in the pulmonary office. He has a BMI of 72. He is suspected to have obesity hypoventilation syndrome (OHS). The pulmonologist is interested in checking his respiratory muscle endurance. Which pulmonary function value can correlate objectively with respiratory muscle endurance measurements?

a. Maximal voluntary ventilation (MVV)
b. FEV1
c. FRC
d. Baseline VO_2
e. Respiratory rate

Correct answer is "a."

MVV can be used as a measure of respiratory muscle endurance. In otherwise healthy obese patients, it may be reduced by 20%. A reduction by 45% may be observed in patients with OHS. Several mechanisms are proposed in this instance. Overstretching of muscle fibers, spine position, and diaphragmatic dysfunction related to increased abdominal fat could be responsible for this effect.

Sharp JT, Druz WS, Kondragunta VR. Diaphragmatic response to body position changes in obese patients with obstructive sleep apnea. Am Rev Respir Dis. 1986;133:32–7.

Investigations for an Obese Patient

Question 5.18

Obese patients generally show poor performance related to high breathing effort tasks when doing pulmonary function tests (PFTs). Maximal voluntary ventilation (MVV) is a test requiring high breathing efforts. Please select the correct statement regarding expected findings in a morbidly obese patient while performing MVV.

a. Slow and deep breathing pattern is observed
b. Relative dead space (VD)/Tidal volume (VT) ratio is increased
c. Relative dead space (VD)/Tidal volume (VT) ratio is decreased
d. Rapid breathing is more economical in terms of O_2 consumption

Correct answer is "b."

In normal subjects, oxygen consumption (VO_2) attributed to respiratory work is less than 3% of the total body consumption of O_2 during quiet breathing. In obese patients, the cost of O_2 may increase to four folds and O_2 consumption increases by 70%. Relative dead space increases and tidal volume tends to fall making the ratio higher.

Koenig SM. Pulmonary complications of obesity. Am J Med Sci. 2001;321:249–79.

Investigations for an Obese Patient

Question 5.19

Select the correct statement about effects of obesity on lung volumes.

a. Expiratory reserve volume (ERV) is increased
b. Expiratory reserve volume (ERV) is decreased
c. Residual volume (RV) is decreased
d. RV to total lung capacity (TLC) ratio is decreased
e. Expiratory reserve volume is increased in supine position

Correct answer is "b."

ERV is likely to be decreased in a morbidly obese patient. This reduction is most observed in supine position. Vital capacity (VC) and total lung capacity (TLC) are usually within normal range in an average obese patient. Residual volume (RV), RV to TLC ratio, resting expenditure of energy, and minute ventilation values are increased. Spirometry shows obstructive effect in severely obese patients. Restrictive effect is seen in mild to moderate forms of obesity.

Ray CS, Sue DY, Bray G, Hansen JE, Wasserman K. Effects of obesity on respiratory function. Am Rev Respir Dis. 1983;128:501–6.

Inselma LS, Milanese A, Deurloo A. Effect of obesity on pulmonary function in children. Pediatr Pulmonol. 1993;16:130–7.

Question 5.20

Carbon monoxide diffusion capacity (DLCO) has a relationship with weight in obese patients. Similarly, a relationship exists between DLCO and alveolar volume. Please select the correct statement regarding this relationship.

   a. Weight loss increases DLCO and DLCO to alveolar volume ratio
   b. Weight gain decreases DLCO and DLCO to alveolar volume ratio
   c. Weight gain increases DLCO and DLCO to alveolar volume ratio
   d. DLCO is inversely related to lung volume measurement
   e. A high DLCO and DLCO ratio is seen in in atelectasis

Correct answer is "c."

DLCO value relates directly to lung volume measurement. High DLCO values are seen in otherwise healthy obese patients. Low DLCO and DLCO to alveolar volume ratio is seen in conditions with loss of pulmonary capillary bed, such as atelectasis.

Ray CS, Sue DY, Bray G, Hansen JE, Wasserman K. Effects of obesity on respiratory function. Am Rev Respir Dis. 1983;128:501–6.

Question 5.21

In healthy subjects, ventilation and perfusion has a specific pattern of distribution. Please select the correct statement.

  a. In normal weight subjects, ventilation is lowest in dependent zones
  b. In obese patients, ventilation may be highest in nondependent zones and there is more perfusion in dependent zones.
  c. In obese patients, perfusion may be predominantly to upper lung zones.
  d. Expiratory reserve volume (ERV) bears no relationship to ventilation perfusion ratio in obese patients

Correct answer is "b."

In otherwise normal subjects, ventilation is highest in dependent lung zones. ERV can be decreased in obese subjects resulting in ventilation shifting to upper zones. Airway closure with alveolar collapse could be the reason for underventilation of lung bases.

Holley HS, Milic-Emili J, Becklake MR, Bates DV. Regional distribution of pulmonary ventilation and perfusion in obesity. J Clin Invest. 1967;46:475–81

Question 5.22

The graphs (Figure 2) reflect information about one of the lung volumes in a normal person and in different clinical situations, including a morbidly obese subject who is otherwise healthy. This lung volume is plotted against time. Looking at the graph, which of the lung volumes is likely shown?

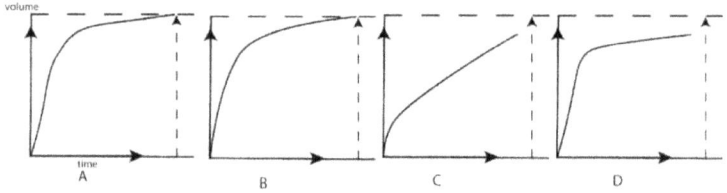

Figure 2

a. Residual volume
b. Forced vital capacity (FVC)
c. Inspiratory reserve volume
d. Tidal volume

Correct answer is "b."

Investigations for an Obese Patient

Question 5.23

Pertaining to the question above, which of the graphs (Figure 2) will be typically seen in a morbidly obese patient who is otherwise healthy.

a. Curve A
b. Curve B
c. Curve C
d. Curve D

Correct answer is "d."

Question 5.24

The patient in the question above is planning to undergo bariatric surgery. His current BMI is 58. Select the correct statement.

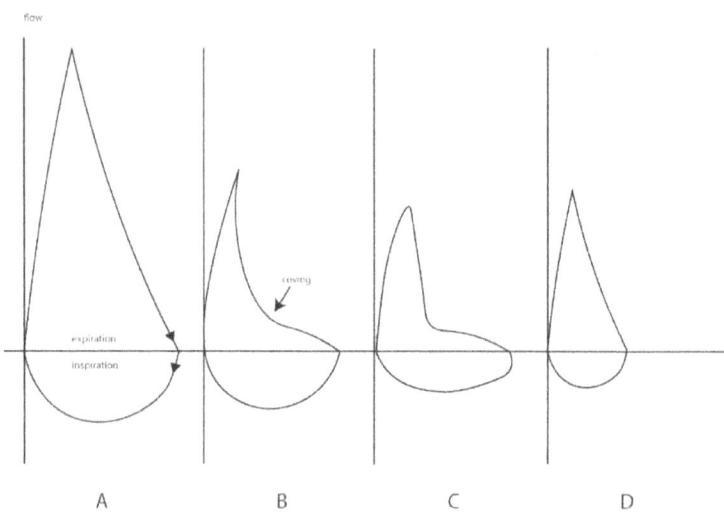

Figure 3

a. His curve of spirometry will more likely be like D
b. His curve of spirometry will more likely be like C
c. Coving seen in the curve is a specific phenomenon seen in morbidly obese patients
d. He is likely to have smaller area under the curve after losing substantial weight

Correct answer is "a."

Investigations for an Obese Patient

Question 5.25

Select the curve (figure 3) which will likely be seen in a morbidly obese patient who loses 95% of excess weight with no history of smoking or bronchial asthma

a. Curve A
b. Curve B
c. Curve C
d. Curve D

Correct answer is "a."
Graph A represents lung function in a typical subject without any respiratory issues. In contrast, Graph B illustrates the relationship in an individual with mild Chronic Obstructive Pulmonary Disease (COPD) featuring an obstructive pattern. As obstructive lung disease progresses, the graph's appearance shifts to resemble Graph C, characterized by the coving effect commonly observed in obstructive airway diseases. Conversely, morbid obesity tends to induce predominantly restrictive effects, maintaining the shape of the loop as depicted in Graph D. Following weight loss post-bariatric surgery, it is anticipated that the area under the curve will likely increase.

Question 5.26

Which of the volumes is affected most in morbid obesity?

a. Td (Tidal volume)
b. TLC (Total lung volume)
c. ERV (Expiratory reserve volume)
d. RV (Residual volume)

Correct answer is "c."
In obese patients, a decrease in Expiratory Reserve Volume is the most seen abnormality. This is thought to be due to decreased functional residual capacity due to the mass loading effect of obesity. TLC and RV are not expected to change much in this situation. Supine position pushes the diaphragm up, leading to fall in ERV.

Ray CS, Sue DY, Bray G, Hansen JE, Wasserman K. Effects of obesity on respiratory function. Am Rev Respir Dis.

Question 5.27

Fat distribution in the body influences pulmonary function. Which of the following is more closely related to adverse effect on pulmonary function?

   a. Abdominal obesity
   b. Obesity of lower extremities
   c. Back
   d. In older people the relationship between distribution of fat pattern and pulmonary function is stronger

Correct answer is "a."

Abdominal obesity is more closely related to pulmonary function abnormality in obese subjects. This effect diminishes with advancing age. It is suggested that abdominal circumference to hip breadth ratio and subscapular skin fold thickness can be objectively related to FEV1 and FVC abnormalities.

Lazarus R, Sparrow D, Weiss ST. Effects of obesity and fat distribution on ventilatory function. Chest. 1997;111:891–8.

Investigations for an Obese Patient

Question 5.28

Pulmonary function test report of an obese patient before bariatric surgery reveals forced vital capacity (FVC) of 2.52 liter (It is 76% of predicted). FEV-1 is 2.09 liters. (78% of predicted) FEV-1/FVC ratio is normal at 83%. FEV (25-75%) is 73% of the predicted value. Slow vital capacity is 2.12 liters (64 % of predicted). Select the correct statement.

a. Report shows mild sleep apnea.
b. Mild obstructive ventilatory defect is present
c. Restrictive disease cannot be ruled out
d. None of the above statements is correct
e. Statements b and c are correct

Correct answer is (e)

The data shown in the question reflects mild obstructive ventilatory defect. The data does not rule out restrictive disease.

Question 5.29

Resting energy expenditure (REE) estimation has a role in understanding and management of obesity. Please select the correct statement about REE / Basal metabolic rate (BMR)

   a. Harris-Benedict equation can be used to assess BMR
   b. Schofield formula is most accurate in assessing BMR
   c. Cunningham's formula gives the best BMR estimations
   d. Indirect calorimetry is the most widely available and used method

Correct answer is "a."

Various formulas including Harris – Benedict equation can be used for the determination of resting energy expenditure. Its accuracy may vary for different BMI ranges. Equipment used to implement indirect calorimetry is expensive and not widely available.

Lee, Sun Hee, and Eun Kyung Kim. "Accuracy of predictive equations for resting metabolic rates and daily energy expenditures of police officials doing shift work by type of work." *Clinical nutrition research* vol. 1,1 (2012): 66-77. doi:10.7762/cnr.2012.1.1.66

Question 5.30

A morbidly obese patient is seen by pulmonologist. Spirometry was done. The report states that forced vital capacity (FVC), FEV1, and FEV1/FVC are normal. There is no significant response to bronchodilator administration. The diffusion capacity is moderately reduced. Expiratory reserve volume (ERV) is reduced and DLCO overcorrects with alveolar volume. The TLC is moderately reduced. Select the correct statement.

    a.   It suggests predominantly obstructive disease.
    b.   It suggests predominantly restrictive disease.
    c.   It suggests neither obstructive nor restrictive disease.
    d.   The facts given are insufficient to comment on obstructive or restrictive disease patterns.

Correct answer is "b."

Restrictive lung disease is commonly seen in morbidly obese patients who are otherwise normal.

Question 5.31

A patient with BMI of 53 is found to have abnormal liver functions. On abdominal ultrasound fatty infiltration of the liver was suspected. A percutaneous core needle liver biopsy was done by the interventional radiologist.

The biopsy demonstrates steatosis score of 2 out of 3. lobular inflammatory score of 3 out of 3 and balloon cells (score 1 of 2). Total score 6 out of 8. A Trichrome stain revealed hepatic cirrhosis (fibrosis stage 4 of 4). The iron stain was negative. A Reticulin stain demonstrates preservation of the reticulin framework. Based on the report stated, select the correct statement.

   a. Patient has steatohepatitis with cirrhosis.
   b. Balloon cells confirm liver cell injury.
   c. Lobular inflammation confirms steatohepatitis.
   d. A score of 0-2 means no nonalcoholic steatohepatitis (NASH).
   e. A score of above 5 is definite NASH.
   f. All above statements are correct.

Correct answer is "f."

Steatosis of less than 5% is scored 0 and more than 66% is scored as 3. Similarly, for ballooning a score of 0 is assigned for no ballooning and 2 is for citing many ballooning cells. For lobular inflammation, a score of 0 to 3 is used. More than 4 foci of inflammation per field is scored as 3. NAFLD activity score (NAS) is determined by combining all the three category scores.

https://www.nature.com/articles/3800680/tables/3 Retrieved on 12/8/2019

Question 5.32

Abdominal ultrasound is requested for a patient with BMI of 57. He has abnormal liver enzymes. AST and ALT were moderately elevated. Fatty liver disease is suspected. Which of the following sonographic findings will be suggestive of fatty liver disease?

 a. Decreased brightness at the surface of liver.
 b. Increased brightness at 4 to 5 cm deep in liver
 c. Hyperechoic 4 to 5 cm deep in liver
 d. Hypoechoic at the surface of liver

Correct answer is "b."

Diagnostic accuracy of NAFLD increases if at least 4 out of 5 sonographic features are present. These include attenuation of image quickly within 4-5 cm of depth, diffuse echogenicity with brightness within the first 2-3 cm of depth, liver being uniformly heterogeneous, thick subcutaneous depth {> 2 cm}, and no visible edges of liver with entire field filled with liver.

Riley TR, Mendoza A, Bruno MA. Bedside ultrasound can predict nonalcoholic fatty liver disease in the hands of clinicians using a prototype image. Dig Dis Sci. 2006;51:982–985.

Question 5.33

Ultrasound of liver is requested for a patient seeking bariatric surgery. Sonography report shows hyperechoic liver. What could be the interpretation with this echo pattern?

   a. Her liver is normal.
   b. Liver has fatty infiltration.
   c. Liver is grossly cirrhotic.
   d. Ultrasound accuracy of picking up fatty liver disease is best when less than 5 % of liver parenchyma is involved with fatty change.

Correct answer is "b."

Hyperechoic image of ultrasound suggests fatty infiltration of liver. Advanced cirrhotic liver may show hypoechoic nodules. Normal liver may contain up to 5% of fat in the parenchyma. Ultrasound is reported to have sensitivity of 84.8% and specificity of 93.6% for diagnosing fatty liver if steatosis is ≥ 20 to 30%.

Hernaez, Ruben et al. "Diagnostic accuracy and reliability of ultrasonography for the detection of fatty liver: a meta-analysis." *Hepatology (Baltimore, Md.)* vol. 54,3 (2011): 1082-1090. doi:10.1002/hep.24452

Question 5.34

Fiberoscan is a test utilized in clinical settings. Select the correct statement.

    a. A test to check clot strength.
    b. A test to check muscle fiber strength.
    c. A test to check fatty liver.
    d. A test to check joint ligaments.

Correct answer is "c."

Ultrasound-based elastography, encompassing shear wave elastography (SWE) and strain elastography, presents noninvasive avenues for evaluating hepatic fibrosis, offering an alternative to traditional liver biopsy. While demonstrating effectiveness in gauging fibrosis and forecasting outcomes in chronic liver ailments, its efficacy in identifying focal liver lesions remains constrained. Variables such as fibrosis, inflammation, blood volume, liver perfusion, fatty infiltration, cholestasis, heart failure, and fasting status influence liver stiffness.

SWE methodologies like transient elastography and point-SWE gauge liver stiffness by measuring shear wave speed, exhibiting commendable diagnostic precision, particularly in chronic hepatitis B and C cases. Transient elastography, extensively researched, showcases robust performance in identifying significant fibrosis and cirrhosis, albeit with optimal cutoff values varying across liver diseases. Yet, challenges arise in obtaining reliable results among obese individuals, those with anatomical irregularities, or hepatic steatosis. Point-SWE and two-dimensional (2D)-SWE utilize acoustic radiation force impulse (ARFI) to produce shear waves for assessing liver stiffness. Point-SWE concurrently displays shear wave speed and ultrasound images, demonstrating comparable diagnostic accuracy to transient elastography. Meanwhile, 2D-SWE generates color-coded elastograms, exhibiting promising sensitivity and specificity in diagnosing liver fibrosis.

Strain elastography, albeit less standardized and quantitative, evaluates tissue strain under stress and may assist in liver fibrosis evaluation. Despite demonstrating moderate diagnostic accuracy, its role remains ambiguous due to limited experience and inter-examiner variability.

Fibroscan, employing a 50-MHz ultrasound wave, estimates liver stiffness in kilopascals (kPa) by measuring shear wave velocity as it traverses liver parenchyma. Stiffness measurements correlate significantly with liver fibrosis and cirrhosis, with Fibroscan boasting nearly 100% sensitivity in detecting cirrhosis compared to the 71% sensitivity of regular ultrasound. Normal stiffness measures range from 2.6 to 6.1 kPa for males and 2.3 to 5.8 kPa for females, with scores exceeding 7.2 kPa suggesting significant fibrosis and those surpassing 14.5 kPa indicating cirrhosis.

https://www.uptodate.com/contents/noninvasive-assessment-of-hepatic-fibrosis-ultrasound-based-elastography?search=fibroscan&source=search_result&selectedTitle=2~54&usage_type=default&display_rank=2

Question 5.35
An ultrasound assessment of the liver was conducted for a patient with morbid obesity. During the examination, the radiologist made a specific observation regarding the liver's echogenicity. Please select the correct statement.

a. Echogenicity is likely to be high.
b. Echogenicity is likely to be low.
c. In fatty liver echogenicity is not altered
d. Routine ultrasound is the best test to comment on liver fibrosis.

Correct answer is "a."

Fatty livers show more echogenicity on sonogram. Fibroscan is a newer high frequency device used in assessing liver stiffness by estimating propagation velocity of a shear wave through liver parenchyma. It can predict liver fibrosis more accurately.

Pathik, Parikh et al. "Fibroscan versus simple noninvasive screening tools in predicting fibrosis in high-risk nonalcoholic fatty liver disease patients from Western India." *Annals of gastroenterology* vol. 28,2 (2015): 281-286.

Question 5.36

Morbid obesity and fatty liver disease are intricately connected. Liver biopsy continues to be a crucial tool in assessing fatty liver disease. The technique used for biopsy can influence pathology findings. Please choose the accurate statement(s) from the following options.

   a. 2 cm or more of the core with at least 11 complete portal tracks are generally considered adequate specimen by most pathologists.
   b. Wedge biopsy is superior to a core biopsy.
   c. Wedge biopsies may under-represent fibrosis.
   d. Prolonged anesthesia time can produce "surgical hepatitis" because of anesthetic gases.
   e. Options "a" and "d" are correct.

The correct answer is "e."

The amount of liver specimen collected, and its location can affect the results. Adequate core biopsy seems to provide enough representative tissue for better interpretation of histopathology. Prolonged anesthesia may cause infiltration of leukocytes resulting in "surgical hepatitis".

Ratziu V, Charlotte F, Heurtier A, *et al.* Sampling variability of liver biopsy in nonalcoholic fatty liver disease. *Gastroenterology* 2005;**128**:1898–1906.

Question 5.37

Differences among pathologists in interpreting liver biopsy specimens for fatty liver are evident. However, there are certain criteria that most experts concur upon. The presence of fat alone or fat along with inflammation and evidence of ballooning are widely accepted criteria. Please choose the correct statement.

a. Fat with inflammation confirms the diagnosis of NAFLD (Nonalcoholic fatty liver disease)
b. Fat with inflammation confirms the diagnosis of NASH (Nonalcoholic steatohepatitis)
c. Fat with inflammation and ballooning confirms the diagnosis of NAFLD
d. Presence of fibrosis in zone 3 (perisinusoidal) points to NAFLD but not NASH

Correct answer is "a."

The presence of ballooning cells qualifies for the diagnosis of NASH. The presence of fibrosis in zone 3 of sinusoids is indicative of past or active NASH.

Question 5.38

Morbid obesity often correlates closely with fatty liver disease. Distinguishing between nonalcoholic fatty liver disease (NAFLD) and alcoholic steatohepatitis (ASH) through liver biopsy can prove challenging in certain instances. However, several distinctions can be discerned through histological examination. Please choose the accurate statement from the options provided.

   a. Mallory hyalines are common in nonalcoholic steatohepatitis (NASH)
   b. Mallory hyalines are common in alcoholic steatohepatitis (ASH)
   c. Neutrophilic infiltrates are more common in NASH.
   d. Foamy degeneration is common in NSAH.

The correct answer is "b."

Mallory hyaline and neutrophilic infiltrates are common histological findings in ASH.

Investigations for an Obese Patient

Question 5.39

Insulin resistance is associated with several distinct effects and associations. It is linked with weight gain and morbid obesity. Please select the correct statement about insulin resistance.

a. Decreased level of C-reactive protein is observed when insulin level is raised.
b. Increased levels of adiponectin are seen in insulin resistance.
c. low-density lipoprotein (LDL) particle size tends to become larger.
d. Decreased atherogenic risk.
e. Intermittent fasting may help reduce insulin resistance.

The correct answer is "e."

Increased level of C-reactive protein, decreased adiponectin, reduced size of low-density lipoprotein particles and increased atherogenic risk are seen with insulin resistance. Beneficial role of intermittent fasting is observed in insulin resistance.

Insulin resistance, characterized by a diminished response to normal insulin levels, holds significant implications in clinical practice due to its association with inadequate glucose response to insulin. Initially identified in diabetic patients requiring increased insulin doses, its definition and clinical importance have evolved over time.

This condition typically results in reduced glucose response to both natural and administered insulin. While often tied to obesity, insulin resistance can stem from various factors including lipodystrophy, stress, medications, pregnancy, genetic anomalies, and autoimmune disorders affecting insulin receptors.

Insulin resistance presents a wide array of clinical symptoms, spanning from metabolic syndrome and abnormal glucose metabolism to cardiovascular issues, kidney disease, skin abnormalities, polycystic ovary syndrome, liver disorders, certain cancers, neurodegenerative diseases, and rare genetic syndromes.

Diagnosing insulin resistance relies heavily on clinical evaluation, particularly in obese individuals exhibiting metabolic syndrome traits like abdominal obesity, high blood sugar, lipid abnormalities, and hypertension. Diagnostic aids include tests measuring serum triglycerides, insulin-to-glucose ratio, and sex hormone-binding globulin, while more sophisticated techniques like euglycemic clamp tests are primarily used in research settings.

Investigations for an Obese Patient

Question 5.40

Which of the following statements about fatty liver is true?

a. Patients with type 1 diabetes have a higher risk of developing fatty liver than patients with type 2 diabetes.
b. Insulin resistance is not a risk factor for developing fatty liver.
c. NASH decreases the risk of hepatocellular carcinoma.
d. ALT level of above 19 in women and more than 30 in men has a high association with fatty liver.

Correct answer is "d."

Patients with type 2 diabetes have a higher risk of developing fatty liver disease. Risk for developing hepatocellular carcinoma is higher with NASH. Insulin resistance is also recognized as a risk factor. High ALT level is correlated with elevated risk of fatty liver.

Investigations for an Obese Patient

Question 5.41

A 47-year-old woman with a history of obesity and well-controlled hypothyroidism presents for a routine follow-up. She reports feeling generally well and mentions that she recently started taking a new multivitamin containing biotin, 10 mg/day, which she has been taking for the past week to improve hair and nail health. Her current medications include levothyroxine 100 mcg daily. Her last thyroid function tests (TFTs) three months ago were within normal limits. During the visit, her physical examination is unremarkable. Routine blood work, including thyroid function tests, is ordered. The results are as follows:

TSH: 0.2 mIU/L (Reference range: 0.4-4.0 mIU/L)

Free T4: 1.0 ng/dL (Reference range: 0.8-2.0 ng/dL)

Free T3: 3.5 pg/mL (Reference range: 2.0-4.4 pg/mL)

Thyroglobulin: 0.5 ng/mL (Reference range: 1.4-78.0 ng/mL)

Given her clinical history and current lab results, what is the most appropriate next step in managing this patient?

   a. Increase her levothyroxine dose to 125 mcg daily due to low TSH.
   b. Repeat the thyroid function tests after stopping biotin for at least 48 hours.
   c. Add liothyronine (T3) therapy to her current regimen.
   d. Order a thyroid ultrasound to assess for thyroid nodules.
   e. ERefer the patient to an endocrinologist for further evaluation.

The correct answer is "b."

The patient's low TSH and normal free T4 and free T3 levels, along with the recent initiation of high-dose biotin supplementation, raise concern for biotin interference in the thyroid function tests. Biotin is known to cause falsely low TSH results and falsely low or high levels of thyroid hormones depending on the assay platform used. The appropriate management in this scenario is to discontinue biotin supplementation and repeat the tests after 48 hours to avoid interference and obtain accurate results. Increasing the levothyroxine dose or adding liothyronine could lead to overtreatment based on inaccurate test results. A thyroid ultrasound or referral to an endocrinologist may be warranted if repeat testing shows persistent abnormalities, but these steps are not appropriate at this time.

Ylli D, Soldin SJ, Stolze B, et al. Biotin Interference in Assays for Thyroid Hormones, Thyrotropin and Thyroglobulin. *Thyroid*. 2021;31(8):1160-1170. doi:10.1089/thy.2020.0866

Principles of Dietary Management

Question 6.1

A morbidly obese patient is suggested to go on a low-carb and low-calorie diet.

Which of the following statements is correct?

    a. A reduction of fasting insulin level is expected

    b. Insulin / Glucagon ratio is likely to increase.

    c. The glycolytic/ lipogenic ratio is increased

    d. Nutritional ketosis is anticipated if dietary intake is 150 to 200 grams of carbohydrates.

    e. In ketosis, dominant fuel for energy is amino acids

The correct answer is "a."

Reduction in insulin level is observed once patients are started on low-carb and low-calorie diets. Nutritional ketosis is seen when 50 gm or less of carbohydrates are ingested per day. Even three to five percent of sustained weight loss is proven to produce significant health benefits, and risks of developing diabetes may reduce by 30% or more.
Phinney, S., Bistrian, B., Wolfe, R., & Blackburn, G. (1983). The human metabolic response to chronic ketosis without caloric restriction: Physical and biochemical adaptation. Metabolism, 32(8), 757-768. doi:10.1016/0026-0495(83)90105-1

5th Edition Principles of Dietary Management

Question 6.2

Patients on low-carb diets develop a state of ketosis. Which of the following statements is correct?

    a. Blood pH is likely to be low with significant metabolic acidosis.

    b. Cardiac and skeletal muscles cannot use ß hydroxybutyric acid and acetoacetic acid as a source of energy.

    c. Decreased activity of hormone-sensitive lipase is expected

    d. Urine output is likely to fall.

    e. Dietary adherence can be checked with breath acetone monitoring.

    f. All the above statements are correct.

The correct answer is "e."

Orthostatic symptoms can appear due to diuresis related to ketone bodies and other mechanisms. The patient may be required to adjust their sodium intake and antihypertensive medications. Similarly, monitoring for gout and blood sugar is needed. Pancreatitis risk is increased if patients with chylomicronemia take low carb and high-fat diets.

Buse, G. J., Riley, K. D., Dress, C. M., & Neumaster, T. D. (2004). Patient with gemfibrozil-controlled hypertriglyceridemia that developed acute pancreatitis after starting ketogenic diet. Current Surgery, 61(2), 224-226. doi:10.1016/s0149-7944(03)00159-4

Question 6.3

A morbidly obese individual with a body mass index (BMI) of 45 is prescribed a low-carb diet to facilitate weight loss. This patient presents with hypertension and obstructive sleep apnea but does not have diabetes. Upon undergoing a urine analysis, ketones are detected. Which of the following statements accurately describes the situation?

   a. It is imperative to limit sodium in the diet.

   b. Renal sodium excretion will be increased

   c. Nutritional ketosis and starvation are similar regarding the loss of lean muscle mass.

   d. Urine output is likely to decrease.

   e. Decreased diuresis is expected in nutritional ketosis.

The correct answer is "b."

Renal sodium excretion tends to increase during ketosis due to several interconnected physiological mechanisms. Firstly, decreased insulin levels in ketosis lead to reduced stimulation for sodium reabsorption in the kidneys, as insulin normally promotes sodium retention. Secondly, increased glucagon levels associated with ketosis oppose the actions of insulin and promote sodium excretion in the kidneys. This occurs through various mechanisms, including the inhibition of sodium reabsorption in the renal tubules. Additionally, ketosis often results in fluid loss through increased urinary output due to the loss of water along with ketones in the urine, contributing to higher sodium excretion. Lastly, ketosis can lead to metabolic acidosis, prompting increased excretion of hydrogen ions in the urine to maintain acid-base balance. This process involves the exchange of sodium ions for hydrogen ions in the renal tubules, further contributing to higher sodium excretion.

Giebisch, G. (2003). Renal potassium transport: mechanisms and regulation. American Journal of Physiology-Renal Physiology, 285(5), F811-F823.

Question 6.4

Low carbohydrate diet produces which of the following effects?

   a. High-density lipoprotein (HDL) levels may rise.
   b. Increased triglycerides.
   c. Significant reduction in low-density lipoproteins (LDL)
   d. A considerable decrease in cholesterol
   e. Weight Watchers, Jenny Craig and Nutrisystem, are typical examples of low carbohydrate diets.

The correct answer is "a."

HDL is expected to be increased with low carbohydrate diets. Triglycerides are likely to be reduced. LDL and cholesterol are not affected significantly. Diets like South Beach and Aitkin are typically considered low carbohydrate diets. Weight Watchers, Jenny Craig and Nutrisystem, are low-calorie diets.

Question 6.5

Low-calorie diets are used as an option for weight loss. Which of the following statements is true regarding low-calorie diets?

a. Nutritional ketosis is observed
b. Cardiac and metabolic risks are reduced
c. Lean muscle mass is likely to be preserved.
d. Examples of low-calorie diets include South Beach and Atkins
e. Low calorie and low carb diets do not have similar cardiovascular risk reductions.

The correct answer is "e."

The low-calorie diets do not produce nutritional ketosis. Their cardiovascular benefits are less pronounced as well. Generally low calorie diet involve monitoring portion sizes, emphasizing whole foods, prioritizing nutrient-rich options, limiting high-calorie foods, balancing macronutrient intake, regularly assessing progress. While low-calorie diets can effectively assist in weight loss and offer health advantages such as improved insulin sensitivity and reduced inflammation, it's crucial to approach calorie restriction cautiously. Overly restrictive diets may lead to nutrient deficiencies, muscle loss, and other adverse effects on health.

Question 6.6

Which of the following statements is true about very low-calorie diets (VLCD)?

a. Daily calories are restricted to 1200 to 1600
b. Very low-calorie diets are available as only prepared formulas.
c. The initial weight loss, especially in the first week, is mainly through loss of body fat
d. VLCDs are very palatable.
e. The natriuresis seen with VLCD is due to insulin reduction and mobilization of liver and muscle glycogen.

The correct answer is "e."

The initial loss of weight is due to diuresis, insulin reduction and moving water with glycogen breakdown. Daily calories are restricted to less than 800 kcal. Diets ranging from 200 to 800 kcal/day are categorized as "very low-calorie diets," while those below 200 kcal/day are termed starvation diets. Although once popular, starvation diets are now discouraged for treating obesity due to their extreme nature and rapid weight loss effects. Very low-calorie diets have not been proven significantly more effective than conventional diets for long-term weight loss. While they may initially lead to greater weight loss, this advantage diminishes over time.

Side effects of very low-calorie diets include hair loss, skin thinning, and an increased risk of gallstones due to the mobilization of cholesterol from fat stores. Pregnant or lactating individuals, as well as children requiring protein for growth, are advised against following these diets.

Very low-calorie diets are best reserved for situations necessitating rapid weight loss, such as before surgery. However, weight regain following discontinuation is common, underscoring the importance of adopting sustainable approaches to weight management.

Tsai, A. G., & Wadden, T. A. (2006). The Evolution of Very-Low-Calorie Diets: An Update and Meta-analysis*. Obesity, 14(8), 1283-1293. doi:10.1038/oby.2006.146

https://www.uptodate.com/contents/obesity-in-adults-dietary-therapy?search=low%20calorie%20diet&source=search_result&selectedTitle=1~137&usage_type=default&display_rank=1

Question 6.7

A morbidly obese patient is enrolled in a medically supervised diet program. A low-calorie and high protein dietary plan was given. Which of the following statements is correct?

   a. Orthostatic symptoms observed may be due to sodium deficiency requiring replacement of sodium.

   b. Gout may precipitate due to a renal mechanism involving competition of uric acid and beta-hydroxybutyric acid in renal tubules.

   c. Diabetic patients need attention and require adjustments in insulin doses with glucose monitoring.

   d. Hypertriglyceridemia of chylomicron origin is a contraindication for low-carbohydrate and high-fat diets.

   e. All the above statements are correct.

The correct answer is "e."

All the above statements are correct. Orthostatic symptoms can appear due to diuresis, and this is seen because of ketone bodies and other mechanisms. Patients may need to adjust to sodium intake and antihypertensive medications. Moreover, monitoring for gout and blood sugar is needed. Pancreatitis risk increases if patients with chylomicronemia take low carb and high-fat diets.

Buse, G. J., Riley, K. D., Dress, C. M., & Neumaster, T. D. (2004). Patient with gemfibrozil-controlled hypertriglyceridemia that developed acute pancreatitis after starting ketogenic diet. Current Surgery, 61(2), 224-226. doi:10.1016/s0149-7944(03)00159-4

Question 6.8

USDA Dietary reference intake (DRI) references protein intake as

    a. 0.1 to 0.5 gm/kg/day

    b. 0.8 to 2.0 gm/kg/day

    c. 3 to 5 gm/kg/day

    d. 6 to 8 gm/kg/day

    e. 9 to 10 gm/kg/day

The correct answer is "b."

Protein requirement is 0.8 to 2.0 gm/kg/day. For fats DRI (USDA) is 30 gm/day

"Read 'Dietary Reference Intakes for Energy, Carbohydrate, Fiber, Fat, Fatty Acids, Cholesterol, Protein, and Amino Acids' at NAP.edu." National Academies Press: OpenBook, www.nap.edu/read/10490/chapter/12.

Question 6.9

A 45-year-old man with a BMI of 32 visits his family doctor for a routine check-up. Upon reviewing his lab results, it's discovered that he has abnormal lipid levels, with elevated LDL and total cholesterol, and low HDL. Additionally, his triglyceride levels are twice the normal range. He was provided with appropriate advice. Please choose the correct statement regarding this scenario.

   a. Reduced dietary intake of fats may lead to an increase in LDL.
   b. Dietary restriction of carbohydrates may lead to a greater decrease in triglycerides.
   c. Reduced dietary intake of fats may lead to a greater decrease of triglycerides.
   d. Dietary restriction of carbohydrates may lead to a greater reduction of LDLs.
   e. A1c and sugar numbers are more related to fat intake rather than carbohydrate intake.

The correct answer is "b."

Triglycerides numbers decrease more once carbohydrates are reduced in the diet. HDL numbers tend to increase. On the other hand, low-fat diets lead to decrease LDL and cholesterol levels. A1c and sugar values are more linked to carbohydrates.

Question 6.10

A patient with morbid obesity is initiated on a very low carbohydrate diet. Please choose the correct option.

   a. Typically, very low carbohydrate means less than 50 grams of carbohydrates.
   b. Very low carb diets generally contain 100 to 150 grams of carbohydrates.
   c. Very low carb containing diets have 160 to 200 grams of carbohydrates.
   d. Very low carb containing diets do not need close supervision of the patient.
   e. Blood pressure is likely to increase in patients on very low carbohydrate containing diets.

The correct answer is "a."

Very low-carbohydrate diets contain less than 50 grams of carbohydrates typically. On the other hand, low-fat diets achieve 10 to 30% of calories from fats. Very low-calorie diets target at below 800 kcal/day. These kinds of diets require medical supervision.

Question 6.11

A morbidly obese patient is enrolled in a dietary regimen that permits her to consume up to 20 grams of carbohydrates initially. She is encouraged to include fish, chicken, and beef in her meals while avoiding processed foods with high glycemic index and those containing trans fats. Which of the following diet plans is most likely to have been chosen in this instance?

   a. Weight watchers
   b. Mediterranean diet
   c. TLC (therapeutic lifestyle change diet)
   d. Atkins diet
   e. Ornish diet

The correct answer is "d."

This dietary plan aligns with the Atkins diet regimen, which encompasses multiple phases, beginning with induction and culminating in a maintenance phase. During the induction phase, individuals are permitted up to twenty grams of carbohydrates, with an emphasis on increased consumption of meats such as beef, chicken, and fish. In the maintenance phase, the allowance for carbohydrates increases to sixty to ninety grams.

In contrast, the Mediterranean diet focuses on natural components like grains, fruits, vegetables, and legumes, while advocating for reduced consumption of processed and high-fat foods, as well as red meats. The Medlife index serves as a valuable tool for monitoring adherence to this dietary program, incorporating factors such as physical activity and social interactions into its scoring system. Additionally, the Mediterranean Diet Adherence Screener (MEDAS) offers another method for assessing adherence to the diet plan.
"How Does a Low Carb Diet Work." Atkins, www.atkins.com/how-it-works.

Question 6.12

A morbidly obese patient with a BMI of 57 undergoes Roux-en-Y gastric bypass surgery for morbid obesity. Following surgery, the patient experiences a leak from the gastrojejunostomy anastomosis and is readmitted. He undergoes abdominal washout in the operating room, and a feeding tube is inserted in the excluded stomach. Subsequently, the patient is managed in the surgical intensive care unit with ventilatory support, and a nutritional consultation is requested.

During the determination of the patient's caloric goals, a discussion takes place with the dietitian. Please choose the correct statement regarding the caloric needs of the patient.

a. 22 to 25 kcal/kg of adjusted body weight
b. 11 to 14 kcal/kg of actual body weight
c. 22 to 25 kcal /kg of actual body weight
d. 22 to 25 kcal/kg of ideal body weight
e. 11 to 14 kcal/kg of ideal body weight
f. BMI can be used as the best index to calculate calories in this case.

The correct answer is "d."

The correct choice in this scenario is option "d."

Obesity is prevalent in ICU settings, affecting up to 75% of patients. Despite appearing to have ample nutritional reserves, critically ill obese individuals are still susceptible to malnutrition. Surprisingly, 57% of hospitalized adults with a BMI exceeding 25 kg/m2 exhibit signs of malnutrition. Obese patients often face challenges in utilizing energy efficiently and are prone to losing lean body mass due to protein metabolism. Mortality rates follow a U-shaped curve concerning BMI, with the highest risk observed in individuals with Class III obesity (BMI > 40 kg/m2) and those with a BMI below 25 kg/m2 (underweight or normal weight). Interestingly, individuals with moderate obesity, with a BMI ranging from 30 to 40 kg/m2, exhibit the lowest mortality rates, a phenomenon termed the obesity paradox.

To mitigate metabolic complications associated with overfeeding and preserve lean body mass, it's recommended to employ a high-protein, hypocaloric feeding approach. In cases where indirect calorimetry (IC) is utilized, the enteral nutrition (EN) regimen should aim for 65-70% of energy requirements across all obesity classes. For patients not undergoing IC, caloric dosing should be tailored based on BMI: 11-14 kcal/kg of actual body weight for BMI of 30-50 kg/m2 and 22-25 kcal/kg of ideal body weight for BMI exceeding 50 kg/m2. Protein recommendations are also based on ideal body weight, with approximately 2.0 g/kg/day recommended for individuals with a BMI of 30-40 kg/m2 and 2.5 g/kg/day for those with a BMI exceeding 40 kg/m2.

"Intensive Care Enteral Nutrition in 2017." Relias Media - Continuing Medical Education Publishing, www.reliasmedia.com/articles/141452-intensive-care-enteral-nutrition-in-2017.

McClave, S A, et al. "Guidelines for the Provision and Assessment of Nutrition Support Therapy in the Adult Critically Ill Patient: Society of Critical Care Medicine (SCCM) and American Society for Parenteral and Enteral Nutrition (A.S.P.E.N.)." JPEN. Journal of Parenteral and Enteral Nutrition., U.S. National Library of Medicine, www.ncbi.nlm.nih.gov/pubmed/19398613.

5th Edition Principles of Dietary Management

Question 6.13

A 45-year-old female patient who is considering joining a commercial weight-loss program. She comes to your office for advice. She has read several testimonials on the program's website, which claim substantial weight loss results. She wants to know how these claims compare to the results from scientific studies and whether he should believe them. Based on recent analyses of weight-loss claims in commercial programs, which of the following statements is most accurate?

a. Testimonials on commercial weight-loss websites are generally aligned with the results from randomized controlled trials (RCTs).
b. Most testimonials on commercial weight-loss websites report typical weight loss outcomes that are supported by scientific evidence.
c. The weight loss claims in testimonials are often greater than those found in randomized controlled trials, and many programs include disclaimers about non-typical results.
d. Only a small fraction of commercial weight-loss programs include any disclaimers about the typicality of the results shown in testimonials.

The correct answer is "c."

A content analysis of 24 commercial weight-loss program websites was conducted to compare their claims to results from randomized controlled trials (RCTs). Researchers reviewed pages and testimonials, abstracting data on demographics, weight loss, and disclaimers. The review found that weight loss claims in testimonials were extreme, with median losses between 10.7 and 49.5 kg, often exceeding results from RCT participants. Only 10 programs had eligible RCTs, and 78% of those included disclaimers noting the non-typical nature of testimonial results. This suggests that commercial testimonials often present higher weight loss than RCT findings, raising questions about the influence of advertising on patient expectations and satisfaction with modest weight loss outcomes.

Vakil RM, Chaudhry ZW, Doshi RS, Clark JM, Gudzune KA. Commercial Programs' Online Weight-Loss Claims Compared to Results from Randomized Controlled Trials. Obesity (Silver Spring). 2017 Nov;25(11):1885-1893. doi: 10.1002/oby.21959. Epub 2017 Sep 2. PMID: 28865085; PMCID: PMC5678966.

Question 6.14

A 35-year-old male patient with obesity is seeking advice on effective dietary interventions for weight loss. He is considering both low-energy diets (LEDs) and very low-energy diets (VLEDs) and wants to understand the differences in outcomes and potential risks associated with each approach. The patient is looking for a dietary plan that will help him lose weight efficiently while also maintaining the weight loss over the long term.

Which of the following statements best describes the outcomes and considerations for low-energy diets (LEDs) and very low-energy diets (VLEDs) in the management of obesity?

a. LEDs typically prescribe less than 800 kcal/day and are suitable for long-term use without medical supervision.

b. VLEDs result in more rapid short-term weight loss compared to LEDs, but both approaches show similar long-term weight loss when combined with lifestyle modification.

c. LEDs induce greater short-term weight loss compared to VLEDs and have a higher participant attrition rate.

d. VLEDs provide a balanced nutrient profile similar to general population recommendations and are free from significant side effects.

The correct answer is "b."

VLEDs, which prescribe less than 800 kcal/day, are associated with faster short-term weight loss but require medical supervision due to potential side effects like cholelithiasis and dehydration. LEDs, typically in the range of 800–1800 kcal/day, offer more moderate weight loss initially. Over the long term, both VLEDs and LEDs, when combined with lifestyle modifications, result in similar weight loss outcomes, although VLEDs produce greater short-term losses.

Chao AM, Quigley KM, Wadden TA. Dietary interventions for obesity: clinical and mechanistic findings. J Clin Invest. 2021 Jan 4;131(1):e140065. doi: 10.1172/JCI140065. PMID: 33393504; PMCID: PMC7773341.

Question 6.15

A 44-year-old female with obesity and type 2 diabetes is seeking dietary interventions to aid in weight loss. She has struggled with self-selected diets in the past and is looking for a simpler, more structured approach to achieve significant weight loss and potentially improve her diabetes management. Which of the following statements best describes the benefits and mechanisms of portion-controlled diets and meal replacements in weight management?

   a. Self-selected diets consistently produce greater long-term weight loss compared to portion-controlled diets.

   b. Portion-controlled diets and meal replacements improve dietary adherence by simplifying meal planning and reducing cognitive demands.

   c. Meal replacements are associated with higher complexity and lower adherence compared to conventional diets.

   d. Portion-controlled diets provide fewer health benefits compared to self-selected diets due to lower initial weight loss.

The correct answer is "b."

Portion-controlled diets, including meal replacements, enhance dietary adherence by reducing the complexity of meal planning, decreasing cognitive demands, and minimizing cues for overeating. These structured approaches lead to greater initial and long-term weight loss compared to self-selected diets. Meal replacements, in particular, support adherence to calorie goals and have been associated with significant health improvements, including diabetes remission in some cases.

Lean ME, et al. Primary care-led weight management for remission of type 2 diabetes (DiRECT): an open-label, cluster-randomised trial. Lancet. 2018;391(10120):541–551. doi: 10.1016/S0140-6736(17)33102-1.

Principles of Dietary Management

Question 6.16

A 40-year-old female patient with obesity is interested in trying intermittent fasting to lose weight. She wants to know how intermittent fasting compares to continuous energy restriction in terms of weight loss and adherence. The patient is looking for a strategy that will be effective for both short-term and long-term weight loss.

Which of the following statements best describes the outcomes and adherence associated with intermittent fasting and continuous energy restriction?

a. Intermittent fasting results in significantly greater long-term weight loss compared to continuous energy restriction.

b. Continuous energy restriction is associated with higher participant adherence and less hunger compared to intermittent fasting.

c. Intermittent fasting and continuous energy restriction result in similar short- and long-term weight loss when isocaloric intakes are prescribed.

d. Participants in intermittent fasting report significantly lower hunger levels and higher adherence compared to continuous energy restriction.

The correct answer is "c."

Studies have shown that intermittent fasting and continuous energy restriction lead to comparable weight loss over short and long terms when caloric intake is matched. While intermittent fasting may address issues like behavioral fatigue and dietary monotony, participant adherence and hunger levels can vary, with some studies noting greater hunger with intermittent fasting at one year.

Beaulieu K, et al. Matched weight loss through intermittent or continuous energy restriction does not lead to compensatory increases in appetite and eating behavior in a randomized controlled trial in women with overweight and obesity. J Nutr. 2020;150(3):623–633.

Question 6.17

A 50-year-old male patient with obesity and impaired glucose tolerance is considering starting a low-fat diet (LFD) to lose weight and improve his health. He is curious about the effectiveness of LFDs compared to other weight loss strategies and wants to understand the potential mechanisms by which LFDs can help him lose weight. Which of the following statements best describes the outcomes and mechanisms associated with low-fat diets (LFDs) in the management of obesity?

a. Low-fat diets generally prescribe more than 30% of calories from fat, making them less effective for weight loss.
b. LFDs have been shown to produce similar weight loss and health improvements as compared to metformin in the Diabetes Prevention Program (DPP).
c. The primary mechanism by which LFDs promote weight loss is through increased satiety due to the higher energy density of fats compared to carbohydrates and proteins.
d. LFDs can lead to significant weight loss by allowing greater food volume intake, which increases satiety and reduces overall energy intake.

The correct answer is "d."

Low-fat diets, typically prescribing less than 30% of calories from fat, have been well-studied and shown to be effective in weight loss and improving comorbid conditions. The Diabetes Prevention Program (DPP) demonstrated that participants on a low-fat diet with caloric restriction lost more weight compared to those on metformin or placebo. LFDs allow greater food volume intake due to lower energy density, increasing satiety and reducing overall energy intake, which contributes to significant weight loss.

Blundell JE, MacDiarmid JI. Fat as a risk factor for overconsumption: satiation, satiety, and patterns of eating. J Am Diet Assoc. 1997;97(7 suppl):S63–S69.

Principles of Dietary Management

Question 6.18

A 50-year-old male patient with obesity and a family history of cardiovascular disease is advised for adopting a Mediterranean diet to help with weight loss and improve his overall health.

His recent laboratory results are as follows:
Fasting glucose: 105 mg/dL (normal: 70-99 mg/dL)
Total cholesterol: 220 mg/dL (normal: <200 mg/dL)
LDL cholesterol: 140 mg/dL (normal: <100 mg/dL)
HDL cholesterol: 45 mg/dL (normal: >40 mg/dL)
Triglycerides: 160 mg/dL (normal: <150 mg/dL)

Which of the following statements best describes the outcomes and mechanisms associated with the Mediterranean diet in the context of weight loss and metabolic health?

a. The Mediterranean diet primarily emphasizes high protein intake, which significantly reduces weight compared to low-fat diets.
b. The Mediterranean diet reduces weight and metabolic abnormalities more effectively when combined with energy restriction and increased physical activity.
c. The Mediterranean diet, when not calorie-restricted, shows significantly greater weight loss than any other dietary interventions.
d. Self-reported adherence to the Mediterranean diet remains consistently high over long-term interventions.

The correct answer is "b."

The Mediterranean diet includes high consumption of vegetables, fruits, legumes, and grains, moderate consumption of red wine and dairy products, and relatively low intake of meat and meat products. Studies have shown that when combined with energy restriction and increased physical activity, the Mediterranean diet results in greater weight loss and metabolic improvements. For example, the DIRECT trial demonstrated stronger effects on weight loss with a calorically restricted Mediterranean diet compared to a low-fat diet. Additionally, the PREDIMED-Plus study showed significant weight loss and improved metabolic health with an energy-restricted Mediterranean diet combined with lifestyle interventions. These benefits make the Mediterranean diet an effective approach for managing weight and reducing cardiovascular risk factors.

Estruch R, et al. Primary prevention of cardiovascular disease with a Mediterranean diet supplemented with extra-virgin olive oil or nuts. N Engl J Med. 2018;378(25):e34. doi: 10.1056/NEJMoa1800389.

5th Edition Principles of Dietary Management

Question 6.19

A 42-year-old female patient with obesity is considering incorporating breakfast into her daily routine to aid in weight loss. She asks whether eating breakfast will help her lose weight and improve her energy intake management. You review recent evidence regarding the impact of breakfast consumption on weight and energy intake. Which of the following statements best describes the findings from randomized controlled trials (RCTs) investigating the effect of breakfast consumption on weight and energy intake?

a. Eating breakfast consistently leads to significant weight loss compared to skipping breakfast.
b. Skipping breakfast results in a small but significant weight loss compared to eating breakfast, with participants who eat breakfast having a higher total daily energy intake.
c. There is no difference in weight loss between individuals who eat breakfast and those who skip it, but breakfast eaters have a significantly lower total daily energy intake.
d. The quality of the studies on breakfast consumption and weight loss is high, with long-term follow-ups providing consistent results.

The correct answer is "b."

Recent meta-analyses of randomized controlled trials (RCTs) found that participants who skipped breakfast experienced a small but significant weight loss compared to those who ate breakfast (mean difference 0.44 kg). Additionally, those assigned to eat breakfast had a higher total daily energy intake (mean difference 259.79 kcal/day). However, the studies included had short-term follow-ups and were at high or unclear risk of bias, suggesting that the findings should be interpreted with caution. Further high-quality RCTs are needed to fully understand the role of breakfast in weight management.

Sievert, K., Hussain, S. M., Page, M. J., Wang, Y., Hughes, H. J., Malek, M., & Cicuttini, F. M. (2019). Effect of breakfast on weight and energy intake: Systematic review and meta-analysis of Randomised Controlled Trials. BMJ, l42. https://doi.org/10.1136/bmj.l42

Question 6.20

A 50-year-old female patient with obesity has achieved a 12% weight loss on a run-in diet. She is now participating in a study that assigns participants to one of three diets based on carbohydrate content (high, moderate, or low) for 20 weeks to maintain weight loss. Her pre-weight loss insulin secretion levels were high. She wants to understand how the carbohydrate content in her diet might affect her energy expenditure and metabolic hormone levels during weight maintenance.

Her recent lab results include:
Fasting glucose: 95 mg/dL (normal: 70-99 mg/dL)
Total cholesterol: 180 mg/dL (normal: <200 mg/dL)
LDL cholesterol: 100 mg/dL (normal: <100 mg/dL)
HDL cholesterol: 50 mg/dL (normal: >40 mg/dL)
Triglycerides: 130 mg/dL (normal: <150 mg/dL)
Fasting insulin: 20 µU/mL (normal: <25 µU/mL)
Which of the following statements best describes the expected outcomes of different carbohydrate content diets on her energy expenditure and metabolic hormone levels?

a. A high carbohydrate diet will result in the highest total energy expenditure and the lowest levels of ghrelin and leptin.
b. A moderate carbohydrate diet will result in higher total energy expenditure than a low carbohydrate diet, with no significant changes in ghrelin and leptin levels.
c. A low carbohydrate diet will increase total energy expenditure and lower ghrelin and leptin levels compared to a high carbohydrate diet, especially in individuals with high insulin secretion.

d. There will be no significant difference in total energy expenditure or hormone levels regardless of the carbohydrate content in the diet.

The correct answer is "c."

In a 20-week controlled feeding trial, participants on a low carbohydrate diet exhibited significantly greater total energy expenditure compared to those on a high carbohydrate diet with similar protein content. Pre-weight loss insulin secretion levels modified individual responses, with higher energy expenditure differences in those with high insulin secretion. The trial's findings support the carbohydrate-insulin model, showing that dietary quality affects energy expenditure independently of body weight. Participants on a low carbohydrate diet had an increase of 209 to 278 kcal/day in energy expenditure, potentially leading to significant long-term weight loss. This effect, consistent with previous studies, suggests a subgroup of individuals may particularly benefit from carbohydrate restriction for obesity treatment.
Ebbeling CB, Feldman HA, Klein GL, Wong JMW, Bielak L, Steltz SK, Luoto PK, Wolfe RR, Wong WW, Ludwig DS. Effects of a low carbohydrate diet on energy expenditure during weight loss maintenance: randomized trial. BMJ. 2018 Nov 14;363:k4583. doi: 10.1136/bmj.k4583. Erratum in: BMJ. 2020 Nov 3;371:m4264. doi: 10.1136/bmj.m4264. PMID: 30429127; PMCID: PMC6233655.

5th Edition Principles of Dietary Management

Question 6.21

A 34-year-old female patient with obesity (BMI 32 kg/m²) has achieved a 12% weight loss on a run-in diet. She is now participating in a study where she is assigned to a high-carbohydrate diet (60% of total energy) for weight-loss maintenance. Her recent lab results are:

Fasting glucose: 90 mg/dL (normal: 70-99 mg/dL)
Total cholesterol: 185 mg/dL (normal: <200 mg/dL)
LDL cholesterol: 110 mg/dL (normal: <100 mg/dL)
HDL cholesterol: 48 mg/dL (normal: >40 mg/dL)
Triglycerides: 135 mg/dL (normal: <150 mg/dL)
Fasting insulin: 18 µU/mL (normal: <25 µU/mL)
Insulin-to-glucagon ratio: 2.5

Considering the carbohydrate-insulin model of obesity, which of the following statements best describes the expected outcomes related to her high-carbohydrate diet?

a. Late postprandial energy availability (EA) will be increased due to higher circulating free fatty acids.
b. Late postprandial energy availability (EA) will be reduced, primarily due to the suppression of free fatty acids, consistent with the carbohydrate-insulin model.
c. The insulin-to-glucagon ratio will decrease significantly, leading to increased late postprandial EA.
d. Early postprandial energy availability (EA) will remain stable, with no significant changes in circulating metabolic fuels.

The correct answer is "b."

According to the carbohydrate-insulin model, a high-carbohydrate diet leads to an elevated insulin-to-glucagon ratio, which directs metabolic fuels toward storage, resulting in lower circulating energy. In a study, the insulin-to-glucagon ratio was significantly higher in participants on a high-carbohydrate diet compared to those on a low-carbohydrate diet. This higher ratio is associated with reduced late postprandial EA, primarily due to the suppression of free fatty acids, which aligns with the carbohydrate-insulin model's predictions.

Shimy KJ, Feldman HA, Klein GL, Bielak L, Ebbeling CB, Ludwig DS. Effects of Dietary Carbohydrate Content on Circulating Metabolic Fuel Availability in the Postprandial State. J Endocr Soc. 2020 May 26;4(7):bvaa062. doi: 10.1210/jendso/bvaa062. PMID: 32666008; PMCID: PMC7326475.

5th Edition Principles of Dietary Management

Question 6.22

A 55-year-old female patient with type 2 diabetes and a BMI of 32 kg/m² presents for a follow-up appointment. She has been following a low carbohydrate, high fat (LCHF) diet for the past 3 months. Her recent lab results are:

A1C: 6.8% (previously 8.1%)
Fasting plasma glucose: 110 mg/dL (previously 153 mg/dL)
Body weight: 80 kg (previously 92 kg)
Total cholesterol: 190 mg/dL (normal: <200 mg/dL)
LDL cholesterol: 120 mg/dL (normal: <100 mg/dL)
HDL cholesterol: 50 mg/dL (normal: >40 mg/dL)
Triglycerides: 130 mg/dL (normal: <150 mg/dL)

Which of the following statements best describes the expected outcomes for the patient following the LCHF diet?

a. The LCHF diet is associated with a minimal change in A1C and body weight, similar to the usual care group.
b. The LCHF diet leads to a significantly greater reduction in A1C and body weight, with more patients discontinuing or reducing antihyperglycemic therapies compared to the usual care group.
c. The LCHF diet results in increased LDL cholesterol levels without significant improvement in glycemic control.
d. The LCHF diet shows no significant difference in fasting plasma glucose levels compared to the usual care group.

The correct answer is "b."

In a study, the LCHF diet was associated with a significant reduction in A1C (−1.29%), body weight (−12.8 kg), and fasting plasma glucose (−43.5 mg/dL) compared to the usual care group. Additionally, all patients initially on insulin therapy in the LCHF group either discontinued it or had a reduction in dose, indicating a metabolically favorable outcome for managing type 2 diabetes.

Ahmed SR, Bellamkonda S, Zilbermint M, et alEffects of the low carbohydrate, high fat diet on glycemic control and body weight in patients with type 2 diabetes: experience from a community-based cohortBMJ Open Diabetes Research and Care 2020;8:e000980. doi: 10.1136/bmjdrc-2019-000980

Question 6.23

A 45-year-old female patient with type 2 diabetes (T2DM) is interested in adopting a low carbohydrate diet (LCD) to manage her condition. She has been struggling with controlling her blood glucose levels and is looking for an effective dietary intervention. Her current medications include metformin and insulin.

Her recent lab results are:

HbA1c: 8.2% (normal: <6.5%)
Fasting glucose: 150 mg/dL (normal: 70-99 mg/dL)
LDL cholesterol: 120 mg/dL (normal: <100 mg/dL)
HDL cholesterol: 45 mg/dL (normal: >40 mg/dL)
Triglycerides: 180 mg/dL (normal: <150 mg/dL)

Considering the findings from a systematic review and meta-analysis, which of the following statements best describes the expected outcomes for the patient following a low carbohydrate diet (LCD) for six months?

a. The patient is unlikely to achieve remission of diabetes or significant weight loss with an LCD.
b. The patient is likely to achieve remission of diabetes (HbA1c <6.5%) and significant weight loss with an LCD, especially if highly adherent, without adverse consequences.
c. The patient will likely experience an improvement in HbA1c without any significant changes in weight or other metabolic parameters.
d. The patient will experience significant improvements in quality of life and LDL cholesterol levels after six months on an LCD.

The correct answer is "b."

A systematic review and meta-analysis of randomized clinical trials indicated that LCDs could lead to higher rates of diabetes remission and significant weight loss at six months compared to control diets. Remission of diabetes was more likely to be achieved when remission was defined as HbA1c <6.5% with or without medication. Significant improvements in triglycerides and insulin sensitivity were also observed. The evidence suggests that patients adhering to an LCD for six months may experience remission of diabetes without adverse consequences, though long-term efficacy and safety remain areas of ongoing research.

Goldenberg JZ, Day A, Brinkworth GD, Sato J, Yamada S, Jönsson T, Beardsley J, Johnson JA, Thabane L, Johnston BC. Efficacy and safety of low and very low carbohydrate diets for type 2 diabetes remission: systematic review and meta-analysis of published and unpublished randomized trial data. BMJ. 2021 Jan 13;372:m4743. doi: 10.1136/bmj.m4743. PMID: 33441384; PMCID: PMC7804828.

5th Edition *Principles of Dietary Management*

Question 6.24

A 45-year-old male with a BMI of 32 kg/m² and a family history of cardiovascular disease (CVD) seeks dietary advice for weight and glycemic control. He has been diagnosed with pre-diabetes and shows signs of insulin resistance. Genetic testing reveals that he carries the APOE4 allele and a high genetic risk score for obesity. He is concerned about the impact of dietary saturated fatty acids (SFAs) on his cardiovascular health and weight management.

Which of the following dietary recommendations is most appropriate for this patient considering his genetic predispositions and current health status?

    a. A diet high in saturated fats and low in carbohydrates to optimize glycemic control and weight management.
    b. A Mediterranean diet rich in unsaturated fats and low in saturated fats, considering his APOE4 allele and risk of cardiovascular disease.
    c. A high-protein diet with moderate carbohydrates and fats, focusing on overall calorie reduction.
    d. A low-fat diet without consideration of carbohydrate intake, primarily to reduce his BMI.

The correct answer is "b."

This patient's genetic predispositions, particularly carrying the APOE4 allele, suggest that he may have a greater fasting plasma lipid response to saturated fat, increasing his risk for cardiovascular disease. Evidence indicates that a Mediterranean diet, which is low in saturated fats and rich in unsaturated fats, can help mitigate this risk by improving lipid profiles and reducing inflammation. Additionally, given his pre-diabetes and insulin resistance, this diet can aid in glycemic control and support weight management without the negative impact of high saturated fat intake. Thus, a personalized dietary approach considering both genetic factors and current health status is essential for optimizing his metabolic health and reducing CVD risk.

Astrup A, Magkos F, Bier DM, Brenna JT, de Oliveira Otto MC, Hill JO, King JC, Mente A, Ordovas JM, Volek JS, Yusuf S, Krauss RM. Saturated Fats and Health: A Reassessment and Proposal for Food-Based Recommendations: JACC State-of-the-Art Review. J Am Coll Cardiol. 2020 Aug 18;76(7):844-857. doi: 10.1016/j.jacc.2020.05.077. Epub 2020 Jun 17. PMID: 32562735.

Question 6.25

A 50-year-old male with a BMI of 30 kg/m² presents with pre-diabetes and a family history of cardiovascular disease (CVD). Recent labs show elevated triglycerides, low HDL cholesterol, and high levels of circulating palmitoleic acid (C16:1). He has been advised to follow a low-carbohydrate diet to manage his insulin resistance and improve metabolic health.

Which of the following statements is most accurate regarding the relationship between dietary saturated fatty acids (SFAs), carbohydrate intake, and cardiovascular risk in this patient?

a. Increased dietary intake of SFAs is directly correlated with higher circulating levels of SFAs and increased cardiovascular risk.
b. Higher carbohydrate intake is associated with increased circulating levels of palmitoleic acid, which correlates with higher cardiovascular risk.
c. Decreased dietary carbohydrate intake leads to increased de novo lipogenesis and higher levels of circulating palmitoleic acid.
d. Saturated fat intake should be minimized in all patients with insulin resistance to reduce the risk of cardiovascular disease.

The correct answer is "b."

In insulin-resistant states, such as metabolic syndrome, pre-diabetes, and type 2 diabetes, there is an increased propensity to convert carbohydrates to fat, leading to elevated levels of circulating saturated fatty acids (SFAs) like palmitoleic acid (C16:1). Elevated levels of palmitoleic acid are strongly linked to obesity, hypertriglyceridemia, hyperglycemia, type 2 diabetes, heart failure, and cardiovascular disease (CVD) mortality. While dietary intake of SFAs does not directly correlate with circulating levels of SFAs, higher carbohydrate intake is associated with increased levels of palmitoleic acid due to enhanced de novo lipogenesis. Therefore, a low-carbohydrate diet can help reduce circulating SFAs and improve metabolic health in patients with insulin resistance.

5th Edition Principles of Dietary Management

Question 6.26

A 45-year-old female with a BMI of 32 kg/m² is referred to a nutritionist for dietary counseling. She has a family history of cardiovascular disease and is concerned about the saturated fat content in her diet. The patient is interested in adopting a low-carbohydrate diet high in saturated fats to manage her weight but is unsure about the health implications.

Which of the following strategies would most effectively address the patient's concerns about saturated fats while promoting overall metabolic health?

a. Advise the patient to avoid all foods high in saturated fats to reduce cardiovascular risk.
b. Educate the patient on the role of whole-fat dairy and other nutrient-dense foods that contain saturated fats in a balanced diet.
c. Recommend a strict low-carbohydrate diet without considering the type and quality of carbohydrates consumed.
d. Emphasize only the reduction of saturated fat intake without addressing the overall quality and type of foods in the diet.

The correct answer is "b."

The long-standing bias against foods rich in saturated fats should be replaced with a more nuanced view that recognizes the importance of the type and quality of fats and carbohydrates consumed. Educating the patient about the role of nutrient-dense foods, such as whole-fat dairy, that contain saturated fats can help meet dietary and nutritional recommendations. Additionally, understanding that low-carbohydrate diets high in saturated fat may improve metabolic health for some individuals can shift focus from simply reducing saturated fat intake to promoting overall dietary quality. Emphasizing culturally sensitive dietary patterns tailored to different populations can further enhance the effectiveness of dietary recommendations.

Astrup A, Magkos F, Bier DM, Brenna JT, de Oliveira Otto MC, Hill JO, King JC, Mente A, Ordovas JM, Volek JS, Yusuf S, Krauss RM. Saturated Fats and Health: A Reassessment and Proposal for Food-Based Recommendations: JACC State-of-the-Art Review. J Am Coll Cardiol. 2020 Aug 18;76(7):844-857. doi: 10.1016/j.jacc.2020.05.077. Epub 2020 Jun 17. PMID: 32562735.

Question 6.27

A 54-year-old male with a BMI of 37 kg/m² and type 2 diabetes mellitus (T2DM) is considering starting a very low-calorie diet (VLCD) to improve his metabolic health. He has a history of hypertension and mild diastolic dysfunction but no other known cardiovascular diseases. His current medications include metformin, lisinopril, and atorvastatin. He presents to the clinic for an evaluation and to discuss the potential benefits and risks associated with VLCD.

Recent laboratory results are as follows:

Fasting glucose: 150 mg/dL
HbA1c: 8.0%
Fasting insulin: 22 µU/mL
HOMA-IR: 6.6
Total cholesterol: 210 mg/dL
HDL cholesterol: 40 mg/dL
LDL cholesterol: 140 mg/dL
Triglycerides: 200 mg/dL
AST: 40 U/L
ALT: 45 U/L

Which of the following statements best describes the expected cardiovascular and metabolic outcomes after 1 week and 8 weeks of a VLCD in this patient?

a. After 1-week, significant weight loss and improvements in insulin resistance are expected, with no changes in liver fat or myocardial triglyceride content.
b. After 1 week, improvements in insulin resistance and reductions in liver fat are expected, but there may be a decrease in myocardial triglyceride content and improvement of cardiac function.
c. After 8 weeks, there will be no significant changes in liver fat or myocardial triglyceride content, but insulin resistance and cardiovascular function will improve.
d. After 8 weeks, significant reductions in liver steatosis, visceral fat, and myocardial triglyceride content are expected, along with improvements in insulin resistance and improvement of cardiac function.

The correct answer is "d."

1 Week: VLCDs are associated with significant metabolic improvements even within the first week, including reductions in liver fat and improvements in insulin resistance (as indicated by decreases in HOMA-IR). However, there is a transient increase in myocardial triglyceride content, which can lead to temporary worsening of cardiac function, including systolic and diastolic function, and increased aortic stiffness.

8 Weeks: With continued adherence to the VLCD, substantial metabolic benefits are observed, including further reductions in liver steatosis and visceral fat. Additionally, myocardial triglyceride content decreases, leading to normalization or improvement of cardiac function. These benefits suggest that VLCDs can be a therapeutic intervention for improving diastolic dysfunction in obesity and diabetes over a longer period.

Taylor, R., et al. (2018). "Mechanism of reversal of type 2 diabetes after bariatric surgery or low-calorie diet: Impact on beta-cell function and insulin sensitivity." Diabetes Care, 41(3), 419-428.

Question 6.28

A 45-year-old male with a BMI of 32 kg/m² and a history of hypertension and type 2 diabetes is seeking advice on effective weight loss strategies. He is interested in trying time-restricted eating (TRE) and wants to know if it would offer better outcomes compared to daily calorie restriction alone.

Which of the following is the most accurate statement regarding the efficacy of time-restricted eating compared to daily calorie restriction for weight loss and metabolic risk factors?

a. Time-restricted eating leads to significantly greater weight loss and improvement in metabolic risk factors compared to daily calorie restriction.
b. Time-restricted eating and daily calorie restriction result in similar weight loss and metabolic outcomes, with no significant difference in efficacy.
c. Time-restricted eating is associated with more adverse events compared to daily calorie restriction.
d. Time-restricted eating should not be considered as a weight loss strategy due to its ineffectiveness.

Correct Answer: B. Time-restricted eating and daily calorie restriction result in similar weight loss and metabolic outcomes, with no significant difference in efficacy.

Comparing time-restricted eating (TRE) with daily calorie restriction revealed that both methods led to similar weight loss and improvements in metabolic risk factors over 12 months. The mean weight loss was not significantly different between the TRE and daily calorie restriction groups, and secondary outcomes, including changes in waist circumference, BMI, body fat, and metabolic risk factors, showed no significant differences. Both approaches were safe, with no notable differences in the number of adverse events between the groups. Consequently, TRE did not provide additional benefits over daily calorie restriction for weight loss or metabolic health.

Liu D, Huang Y, Huang C, Yang S, Wei X, Zhang P, Guo D, Lin J, Xu B, Li C, He H, He J, Liu S, Shi L, Xue Y, Zhang H. Calorie Restriction with or without Time-Restricted Eating in Weight Loss. N Engl J Med. 2022 Apr 21;386(16):1495-1504. doi: 10.1056/NEJMoa2114833. PMID: 35443107.

Role of Physical Activity in Management of Obesity

Question 7.1

Which of the following statements is true regarding the need for physical activity in weight maintenance?

a. People doing 150 to 250 minutes of moderate intensity physical activity per week are likely to have a stable weight profile.

b. A steady weight is regarded as up to 10-15% of the change in body weight over the length of time.

c. Physical exercise alone can be a useful strategy for most people to lose significant weight.

d. Significant fluctuations in weight are not associated with an increased risk of cardiovascular disease and all-cause mortality.

e. The guidelines issued by various organizations do not vary considerably in the amount of physical activity needed to have a stable weight profile.

The correct statement is "a."

30 to 60 minutes of daily moderate-intensity exercise for five days in a week or vigorous-intensity exercise three times a week is recommended. Considerable variation in guidelines by various organizations exists.

Donnelly, J. E., Blair, S. N., Jakicic, J. M., Manore, M. M., Rankin, J. W., & Smith, B. K. (2009). Appropriate Physical Activity Intervention Strategies for Weight Loss and Prevention of Weight Regain for Adults. Medicine & Science in Sports & Exercise, 41(2), 459-471. doi:10.1249/mss.0b013e3181949333

Question 7.2

Which of the following statements is correct about MET (Metabolic Equivalent), exercise prescription and stress testing?

a. MET is the amount of oxygen consumed or metabolic work done during slow walking, and it is equal to 1 MET.

b. Walking at four mph on a level and firm surface is considered 2 METS.

c. A minimum exercise prescription should contain five components including frequency, intensity, time, type, and specific precautions.

d. Nuclear imaging stress testing can be done easily for all weight ranges.

e. None of the above statements is correct.

The correct statement is "c."

The amount of oxygen consumed, or metabolic work done during quiet sitting is considered 1 MET. Light physical activity is < 3 METs. Moderate exercise is 3-6 METS, and vigorous activity is > 6 METs. Standing takes 2 METs.

Pate, R. R. (1995). Physical Activity and Public Health. Jama, 273(5), 402. doi:10.1001/jama.1995.03520290054029

Question 7.3

NEAT is an acronym for non-exercise activity thermogenesis. Which of the following statements is correct about NEAT?

a. Non-exercise related energy expenditure can be up to 2000 kcal.

b. Increasing standing or ambulation time by 2.5 hours every day may result in spending up to 350 kcal additionally.

c. Higher NEAT may lead to a decrease in the required amount of heavy exercise target of suggested 300 minutes in a week.

d. Climbing stairs can range between 5 to 8 METs of activity.

e. All the above statements are correct.

The correct statement is "e."

All the above statements are correct. NEAT's role may establish as more data becomes available. Replacing sedentary behaviors with active lifestyle and activity may help in weight maintenance.

Black AE, Coward WA, Cole TJ, Prentice AM: (1996). Human energy expenditure in affluent.

Question 7.4

Which of the following statements accurately reflects the impact of adding exercise to diets with moderate to severe caloric restriction in moderately overweight adults?

a. Exercise significantly enhances weight loss and is essential for achieving substantial reductions in body weight.
b. Adding exercise to caloric restriction has only a minimal effect on weight loss but may offer additional benefits independent of weight loss, such as attenuating the loss of muscle mass.
c. Exercise programs combined with caloric restriction lead to substantial weight loss, particularly when individuals are moderately overweight.
d. The addition of exercise to caloric restriction results in minimal weight loss and does not provide any additional benefits beyond calorie restriction alone.

The correct statement is "b."

For moderately overweight adults, incorporating exercise into diets with moderate to severe caloric restriction results in minimal weight loss impact. Nonetheless, exercise offers significant advantages beyond simply reducing weight. It assists in maintaining muscle mass, counterbalances the decline in energy expenditure during weight loss, and facilitates adherence to necessary calorie restrictions. These aspects are particularly crucial when utilizing potent anti-obesity medications or undergoing bariatric surgery, as substantial weight loss may heighten worries about lean body mass loss.

https://www.uptodate.com/contents/obesity-in-adults-role-of-physical-activity-and-exercise?search=obesity%20and%20physical%20activity&source=search_result&selectedTitle=1~150&usage_type=default&display_rank=1#H27963546

Question 7.4

Which of the following statements accurately reflects the findings regarding exercise and weight loss?

a. Progressive resistance strength training is ineffective for improving physical functioning in older adults.
b. In studies involving individuals with obesity, aerobic exercise alone was found to be the most effective for weight loss and health improvements.
c. Combined aerobic and resistance training has minimal impact on cardiorespiratory fitness and abdominal fat reduction.
d. Walking is not considered an appropriate form of exercise for weight loss, and structured aerobic activities are always superior in effectiveness.

The correct statement is "b."

The most effective combination of aerobic and resistance exercises remains uncertain. Evidence suggests that progressive resistance strength training enhances physical functioning among older adults. In a study involving individuals with obesity, those assigned to resistance, aerobic, or combined exercise groups experienced weight loss and improvements in various health indicators compared to a sedentary control group. Combined aerobic and resistance training yielded the most significant benefits, improving cardiorespiratory fitness, reducing abdominal fat, increasing endurance, and enhancing insulin sensitivity. Walking is considered a suitable form of exercise for many individuals, with research indicating its effectiveness for weight loss when combined with dietary adjustments and incorporating brief periods of activity into daily routines.

Role of Physical Activity in Management of Obesity

Question 7.5

A 75-year-old sedentary woman resident of a senior living home, with a BMI of 37 kg/m² is concerned about her mobility and the risk of developing major mobility disability (MMD), defined as the inability to walk 400 meters. She is considering participating in a structured physical activity (PA) program. Based on the Lifestyle Interventions and Independence for Elders (LIFE) Study, which tested the effects of a moderate-intensity PA intervention versus a health education (HE) program on mobility among older adults, what is the most likely outcome for her if she participates in the PA program?

   a. The PA intervention will have no significant impact on her risk of developing MMD.
   b. The PA intervention will increase her risk of developing MMD compared to the HE program.
   c. The PA intervention will reduce her risk of developing MMD, but the effect will be less significant than in non-obese participants.
   d. The PA intervention will reduce her risk of developing MMD, with a notable benefit observed even in those with extreme obesity (class 2+ obesity).

The correct statement is "d."

The LIFE study found that a structured PA program significantly reduced the risk of major mobility disability (MMD) in older adults, including those with class 2+ obesity (BMI ≥ 35 kg/m²). The hazard ratio (HR) for participants with class 2+ obesity was 0.69, indicating a 31% reduction in the risk of MMD compared to those not participating in the PA program. This suggests that despite the challenges associated with extreme obesity, a structured PA program can offer substantial benefits in maintaining mobility and reducing the risk of disability in older adults. The study did not find a statistically significant difference in the benefit of the PA intervention across different obesity categories, emphasizing the efficacy of PA in improving mobility regardless of baseline obesity status.

Question 7.6

A 55-year-old male with a BMI of 37 kg/m² presents to your clinic seeking help with weight loss. He has no history of diabetes but has struggled with obesity for many years. He has completed an 8-week low-calorie diet, resulting in a weight loss of 12% of his initial body weight. He is interested in maintaining this weight loss and further improving his health. Which strategy is most likely to lead to the greatest weight loss, reduction in body-fat percentage, and additional health benefits over one year?

  a. Exercise program
  b. Liraglutide (3.0 mg per day) plus usual activity
  c. Exercise program plus liraglutide therapy
  d. usual activity

The correct statement is "c."

In a randomized, head-to-head, placebo-controlled trial, adults with obesity who did not have diabetes were assigned to four strategies after an 8-week low-calorie diet: exercise plus placebo, liraglutide plus usual activity, exercise plus liraglutide, and placebo plus usual activity. After one year, the combined exercise and liraglutide group showed the greatest weight loss and reduction in body-fat percentage, achieving a 16% total weight loss, along with significant improvements in glycated hemoglobin levels, insulin sensitivity, cardiorespiratory fitness, and overall well-being. This combination was more effective than either treatment alone or placebo.

Lundgren JR, Janus C, Jensen SBK, Juhl CR, Olsen LM, Christensen RM, Svane MS, Bandholm T, Bojsen-Møller KN, Blond MB, Jensen JB, Stallknecht BM, Holst JJ, Madsbad S,

Torekov SS. Healthy Weight Loss Maintenance with Exercise, Liraglutide, or Both Combined. N Engl J Med. 2021 May 6;384(18):1719-1730. doi: 10.1056/NEJMoa2028198. PMID: 33951361.

Question 7.7

A 45-year-old female who has successfully maintained a weight loss of 35 lbs for over a year is part of the National Weight Control Registry. She engages in regular physical activity and is interested in optimizing her exercise routine for long-term success. Which of the following strategies is associated with the greatest benefit in maintaining high levels of moderate-to-vigorous physical activity (MVPA) and exercise habit strength?

a. Engaging in exercise at varying times throughout the week to avoid monotony.
b. Consistently exercising in the early morning at least 50% of the time.
c. Focusing solely on the intensity of exercise rather than the timing.
d. Participating in evening exercise sessions due to fewer distractions.

The correct statement is "b."

Consistent exercise, especially in the early morning, is associated with greater MVPA levels, stability in exercise routines, and higher exercise automaticity (habit strength) over time. Consistent morning exercise may help establish a regular routine due to fewer scheduling conflicts and can reinforce habit formation, making it easier to maintain regular physical activity. This approach contrasts with varying exercise times, which may disrupt the establishment of a consistent routine and reduce overall physical activity levels.

Schumacher LM, Thomas JG, Wing RR, Raynor HA, Rhodes RE, Bond DS. Sustaining Regular Exercise During Weight Loss Maintenance: The Role of Consistent Exercise Timing. *J Phys*

Act Health. 2021;18(10):1253-1260. Published 2021 Aug 14. doi:10.1123/jpah.2021-0135cal activity levels.

Book Page

https://www.facebook.com/MedicalFronts

For List of Errata Visit

https://obesityreviewmultiplechoicequestions.blogspot.com/2019/01/obesity-qeustions.html

Obesity Insights and Learning: Self-Assessment Exam

(Another resource to practice obesity questions)

https://medicalfronts.com/index.php/obesity-insights-and-learning/

www.ingramcontent.com/pod-product-compliance
Lightning Source LLC
Chambersburg PA
CBHW052147220526
45471CB00004B/1560